D1231968

DEMCO

The
Kamasutra
for Women

Also available in English, by Vinod Verma:

Ayurveda: A Way of Life
Ayurveda for Life

The
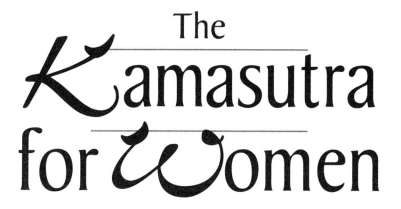

Kamasutra
for Women

THE MODERN WOMAN'S WAY
TO SENSUAL FULFILLMENT
AND HEALTH

Vinod Verma

KODANSHA INTERNATIONAL

New York • Tokyo • London

Kodansha America, Inc.
575 Lexington Avenue, New York, New York 10022, U.S.A.

Kodansha International Ltd.
17-14 Otowa 1-chome, Bunkyo-ku, Tokyo 112, Japan

Published in 1997 by Kodansha America, Inc.
by arrangement with the author.

Originally published in German translation in 1994 under the title *Kamasutra für Frauen* by Scherz Verlag, Bern. German translation copyright © 1994 by Scherz Verlag.

Figures 2, 4–27, and 29–34 were drawn by Phyllis Palmer. Figures 1, 3, 28, and 35 by Nancy B. Field.

Credits for paintings and sculptures can be found in the List of Paintings and Sculptures on p. xi.

Library of Congress Cataloging-in-Publication Data
Verma, Vinod, 1947–
    [Kamasutra für Frauen. English]
    The Kamasutra for women : the modern woman's way to sensual
fulfillment and health / Vinod Verma.
      p. cm.
    ISBN 1-56836-141-6
    1. Sex instruction for women.   2. Women–Sexual behavior.
3. Vātsyāyana. Kamāsutra. I. Title.
HQ46.V4513   1997
306.7'082—dc21   97-26171
                                        CIP

Printed in the United States of America

05 04 03 02   10 9 8 7 6 5 4 3 2

Dedicated to all those men who accept
the eternal female within themselves
and love and respect women
as their mothers, sisters,
companions, and daughters.

Even an outrageous man
should not be harsh to a woman
remembering that
upon her, depends the joy of sensuous love,
pleasure and virtue.
A woman is an ever holy field,
in which the Self is born.
Even the sages do not possess the power
to procreate without her.
—*Mahabharata*
I (74), 51–52

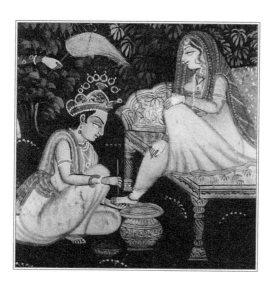

Contents

$\mathcal{L}$ist of Paintings and Sculptures

Disclaimer

The information provided in this book is not intended in any way to replace the services of a physician, but to educate readers about alternative remedies in the interest of increased health awareness. Neither the author nor the publisher makes any specific medical claims for the recipes and remedies presented herein. The suggestions in this book should be undertaken only under the guidance or supervision of a doctor or other appropriate health professional. Please consult a doctor for any problems you may be having.

$\mathcal{A}$ Word about the Hindi and Sanskrit in This Book

Out of respect for the conventions of classic Indian literature, each of the eleven sutras of the eleven parts of this book, as well as the ritual conclusions to each part, are given in both English and Hindi, the modern outgrowth of Sanskrit.

In the interest of the general reader, the Sanskrit words that occur in the English text are translated according to their approximate pronunciation in English.

*P*reface to
the English Edition

Ever since I finished writing this book, I have been lecturing and giving seminars on this theme to mixed groups, as well as exclusively to women in Germany and Switzerland. Women have shown a great enthusiasm for this kind of group meeting where they were able not only to learn recipes for certain health problems or rejuvenate their sexual energies but also to share experiences with each other, learn to be strong and courageous, and develop the ability to find reasons behind their problems.

It is remarkable how many men told me that this work helped them to understand women's sexual reactions and to develop better relationships at many levels of existence. However, several men also complained that the book did not deal specifically with their problems. I admit this drawback and am preparing a volume on "eternal male energy," in which I will attempt to provide some answers to many of the issues men raised in my seminars or otherwise.

At times, I have also had to face hostility from some persons who felt that it is presumptuous for me to write and talk about women's freedom, strength, and sexuality, since I come from a "Third World country where women are tortured." These are the people whose entire range of knowledge of India, its culture, and Indian women has come through sensationalist reports about burning brides. In any event, I do not propose this book as a solution to criminal problems, whether in India or elsewhere.

The problems of women discussed in this book do not restrict themselves to any particular country or community or religion. They are fundamental problems concerning women globally. My organization and I have researched these questions extensively to assure that the study is both wide-ranging and original. I have purposely left out problems limited to a particular country or group.

The title of this book confused some German and Swiss reviewers who in response termed the *Kamasutra of Vatsyayana* the "Kamasutra for men." I feel strongly that the title of this ancient book of wisdom should not be distorted. *The Kamasutra for Women* is not an altered version of the classical Kamasutra; it is an entirely different book which, for the first time, focuses on profound aspects of sexuality from a holistic and woman's point of view, and especially deals with women's sex-related health problems.

Sexual energy is a very powerful source of energy, and it should be channeled properly. When it is suppressed, misguided, or misused, it can give rise to serious, even fatal health problems. It can also create social imbalances, thus paving the way for eventual social crises. To give sexuality a positive and beneficial direction, we need first to acknowledge it, not treat it as some kind of snack entertainment, as if it were equivalent to munching on popcorn or potato chips.

Preface

A little less than two thousand years ago, in the land presently known as India, a great treatise was written on *Kama*, sensuous love, by the sage Vatsyayana. The treatise was written in the form of aphorisms, or *sutras*—thus the name, *Kamasutra*. According to the Hindu holistic way of looking at life, a sexual and love relationship between a man and a woman cannot be visualized independent of the social, psychological, and spiritual context in which it occurs. Everything in this universe is interdependent and interconnected. Our way of living, our health, our immediate circumstances, our beliefs, rituals, and social customs directly affect our sexuality; and our sexual expression influences our own equilibrium and well-being. All these things were taken into consideration by Vatsyayana.

Although for convenience *Kama* is often translated as "sexuality," it in fact denotes "sensuality" in its totality, which means the feelings and expressions of pleasure and pain deriving from all five senses. The senses are in turn governed by the mind—itself constantly undergoing modification through the senses. But the mind is also capable of going beyond sensuality; when we bring it to a state of stillness, it withdraws from the senses and stops modifying. In this unmodified state, the human experience is beyond the sensuous, and the mind becomes one with the soul or spirit. The soul never modifies; like a reflecting glass, it reflects the activities of the mind and is the cause of consciousness.[1]

Desire for worldly pleasures arises from the senses. The root word *Kama* can be readily identified in the word for "desire," *kamana*. When we use the word *Kama*, we mean much more than simple sexuality or sexual pleasure. Sexuality is one among a million other sensuous experiences, and cannot be treated exclusively and independently. In ancient India, sexuality was integrated within the body of written and figurative expression. A. L. Basham, in his famous book *The Wonder That Was India*, wrote: "The literature of Hindu India, both religious and secular, is full of sexual allusions, sexual symbolism, and passages of frank eroticism. . . . The erotic preoccupations of ancient India are made very evident in art and literature."[2]

Unlike Western scholars, I would say that ancient Indians were not so much "preoccupied" by erotics as they were accepting of sexuality as an integrated part of life, along with other sensuous experiences. Sexuality was not compartmentalized and treated exclusively, nor considered demanding of seclusion and secrecy. This is hardly surprising, since the ancient Indians viewed the universe as a perfectly organized whole which is ever changing and dynamic, where nothing happens fortuitously and everything is interconnected, interrelated, and interdependent.

The most ancient books from India are the four Vedas, or books of wisdom, which were written at least thirty-five hundred years ago. In the *Atharva Veda*, lust is praised as follows:

> *Lust was born first: neither gods, nor ancestors, nor men*
> *can equal him. Oh lust! you are immense as you reside in all*
> *living beings. I bow to you. You are a higher deity than the*
> *sun, moon, wind, fire. You are assimilated in all and,*
> *therefore, you are forever great, I bow to you.*[3]

The union of male and female holds a sacred place in Indian tradition. It symbolizes the union and dissolution of two principal cosmic energies and complementary forces which give rise to a feeling of a unique bliss. The combination of the *Purusha*, or Universal Soul, with the *Prakriti*, or Cosmic Substance (see Part II), is the cause of the phenomenal world, and their complete dissolution into each other paves the way for ultimate freedom and immortality. The momentary physical joy of sexual union can be prolonged and extended to a spiritual and cosmic experience—but only if we try to see life in its totality and our relationship to the cosmic system.

So why another Kamasutra? And why a Kamasutra for women? I have two principal reasons for this new effort. First, the sage Vatsyayana wrote his treatise at a time when there was a holistic approach to life. People of his age did not live, as we do, in a fragmented way, segregating the physical, psychological, social, economical, sexual, and spiritual aspects of their lives. I believe we need another Kamasutra to address the new ways of life and changing times, to bring into modern social consciousness the holistic way of life, and to demonstrate that sexuality is not merely a fragment of our existence but a part related and linked to all other aspects of our lives.

Second, the author of the original Kamasutra was a man, and he addressed his book largely to men. His descriptions of women represent an outsider's point of view. I believe we need to look at sexuality also from the viewpoint of women and to go into the details of the problems related to their sexuality, including their major physiological and psychological changes.

The beginning and end of menstruation, pregnancy, and childbirth are major events that directly affect a woman's sexual vigor and energy. In giving birth, she undergoes the pains and perils of creation; later a tremendous amount of energy and effort is devoted to motherhood. A woman needs to learn to handle various aspects of her femininity efficiently so that her sexual expression remains undisturbed and her sexual energy flows unhindered. This book is meant to provide her a guide in this direction, while at the same time inspiring her male partner to understand her better.

India's ancient medical literature, as well as its present-day living tradition, contains a great deal of wisdom concerning women. Unfortunately, this wisdom is scattered here and there, and due to rapid industrialization, the oral tradition is slowly getting lost. I have attempted to compile all this wisdom in one place for the worldwide benefit of "womankind" and ultimate benefit of "mankind." Pleasure, happiness, and intensity of experiences in human life depend upon our physical well-being, which depends upon our inner and outer equilibrium.

A woman is the nucleus of a family system. This gives her more responsibility than her male partner. On the other hand, she needs more care and more attention, understanding, and indulgence from her partner because of her ever-changing physical and psychological state and the extra responsibility of creation and motherhood. This book is meant to help self-aware men better understand the various dimensions of a woman's sexuality and to point them towards more balanced, harmonious, and fulfilling relationships with their female companions. The last six Parts of the book on sexual interaction are equally important for both sexes.

Movements for women's liberation from the conservative, narrow vision of their role have gained impetus in recent years, as women have raised their voice against past exploitation. This book is written with similar views. It aims to lead women to self-assurance and strength. Women are not passive social partners for men, nor in any way inferior in their sexual participation. They are also not "equal" to men, and neither can men be "equal" to them; they are both different and complementary to each other. Both men and women are an integral part of each other, and each is incomplete without the other.

We must understand that the exploitation and suppression of women is not necessarily organized and legalized by men. It is rather the whole system which is imbalanced. The solution is not to quarrel with men and blame them for the harm, but to cure the wrongs of our social system. To alter the fundamental philosophical basis of the whole system will require both men and women.

My point of view on this subject is similar to my views on health. There are always infections and diseases around us. By making ourselves stronger, by keeping our physical and mental energies in equilibrium, we can both save ourselves from innate disorders and ward off any external attack. Similarly, I believe that women must make themselves strong in every respect. We (men or women or any social group or nation) must remember that we are exploited when we let ourselves be exploited. Trees which have deep roots do not fall easily in a storm; their roots have expanded in a profound part of the earth.

The theoretical basis of this book is provided by the fundamental ideas of cosmic unity propounded by various schools of thought in ancient India and, specifically, the principles of the Sankhya speculative school of thought, which provide the metaphysical basis for the disciplines of yoga and Ayurveda (the ancient Indian science of life). For a deeper comprehension of this thought beyond what is possible to present in this book, the reader is advised to see the introductory chapters of my other books on yoga or Ayurveda, or to go back to the ancient books themselves. Practical aspects of this book are derived from yogic, Ayurvedic, and ethnic wisdom, as well as research carried out in the context of our modern technologically oriented life.

The book treats eleven major themes in eleven Parts. Each Part contains eleven sutras in Hindi and English, explanations in English, and, where appropriate, further philosophical or practical elaboration on aspects of the theme, including herbal and homeopathic recipes and yogic exercises.

I have chosen to write this book in the form of aphorisms, or sutras, not because of the well-known *Kamasutra of Vatsyayana* but because I am greatly influenced by this ancient writing style. In India, this style was adopted more than three thousand years ago when the ceremonial prescriptions were reduced to a more compact form and to a more precise and scientific system. The book which has influenced me the most is the *Yoga Sutra of Patanjali*, which I have translated, with commentary.[4] Patanjali wrote his yoga sutras around the fifth century B.C. The four parts of the book include 191 sutras in which the great master elucidates in "a mathematical manner" the discipline of yoga, gradually taking you on a journey to your innermost being, which expands into the cosmic reality. Because of this example, I feel that use of aphorisms—expressions of principles in short and pithy sentences so that the principles can easily be remembered—is a very effective way of disseminating practical knowledge.

This book is a part of the multiple efforts made by NOW (The New Way Health Organization) to spread the message of a wholesome living in harmony with our surroundings and the cosmic forces. I founded NOW in 1986 in Germany when I realized that the great health institutes for which I had been doing research for sixteen years were directing almost all their efforts and resources towards disease, not health. I felt the need for an organization that concentrated on holistic health through holistic living.

In human history, women have played a very important role in keeping the age-old values alive which help establish peace and harmony on our globe. I ask the women of the world to develop courage in order to face the forces which disintegrate us and lead us to a fragmented way of living. A woman can undertake and accomplish this task with a greater facility than a man, since his existence begins in her womb.

Dr. Vinod Verma
February 1993–November 1995
NOW (The New Way Health Organization)
Noida, India/Freiburg, Germany

Acknowledgments

I pay my respect and homage to the guru of the gurus, Patanjali, from whom I have learned the style of writing sutras. His deductive clarity and logic helped me to render this theme in a modern form.

I am most grateful to my father, who taught me to develop courage and strength and made me understand that these were the most essential qualities for any success in life. These values helped me fight the toughest situations with ease, and I do not remember a single incident of my life when I had to feel helpless or small because of being a woman. They have made me lead an enriched and fulfilled life without which it would not have been possible to write this book.

I extend my warm thanks to Dr. Kapila Vatsyayan, the academic director of the Indira Gandhi National Centre for the Arts, for her very inspiring discussions. I am also indebted to Dr. N. D. Sharma of the same center for going through the sutras in Hindi.

I express my deep gratitude to the following friends: Mahendra Kulsreshtha for editorial assistance; Eckhard Biermann and Andrea Wolf-Biermann for providing me home as well as office facilities in Freiburg; and Nancy Meyerson-Hess for inspiring discussions, encouragement, and support. I am also indebted to some other friends who helped me in various ways but would not like to have their names mentioned.

For illustrations in this book, I am grateful to my brother Kuldeep (Kuku) for taking yogasana photographs, used as the basis for the drawings in the present edition; to Arun Kundalia for making the computer drawings; and to Prof. Rekha Jhanji, art advisor of our organization, for allowing me to use her miniature paintings from her private collection. I am grateful to the Archeological Survey of India for providing the photographs of temple sculptures, and to the National Museum, New Delhi, for providing me the picture of the dancing figure from Mohenjadaro.

I have been working on this research project since 1986, and to get an insight into this field, I had to collect information and data from a cross section of society in different communities of various religions, and from various countries. I extend my profound gratitude to all those who shared without hesitation their personal experiences, thoughts, joys, and pains.

I acknowledge my gratitude to Kodansha for bringing out the American edition of this book, and I am thankful to their staff for coordinating and accommodating my odd schedules.

The
Kamasutra
for Women

PART I
Self-Awareness

. . .

पहला भाग
नारीत्व का बोध

. . .

What is that what a poet can not observe?
What is that what a woman can not do?
What is that what a drunken can not say?
What is that what a crow can not eat?

—*Canakya*

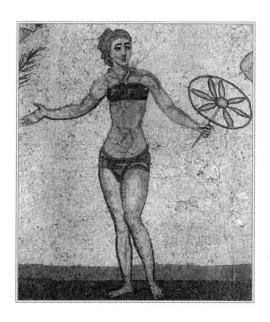

१. इस ग्रन्थ की रचना स्त्री और पुरुष दोनों के उपयोग के लिए तथा अनुकूल वातावरण उत्पन्न करने के लिए की जा रही है।

1. **This book is written for the benefit and fulfillment of men and women, and to help create a harmonious social environment.**

Though this book is titled *The Kamasutra for Women*, its contents are meant to educate both men and women about the multiple aspects of a woman's life and various facets of her sexuality. A woman needs to know herself and comprehend the biological changes that affect her life and emotional state. If she does not make an effort to live in harmony with the major events in her life like pregnancy, childbirth, and lactation, her health deteriorates, she feels frustrated, and her sexual energy is severely hindered.

A woman's immediate social environment is generally her male partner. He equally needs to learn about a woman's body, mind, and inner needs. If he lacks an understanding of women in general, he cannot understand his female partner in particular. Misunderstandings will arise, leading to sexual imbalance, which may become the root cause of disharmony between the two and give rise to further problems with others. This imbalance in the smallest social unit, the family, will bring unpleasant consequences for the children, and many such troubled families lead to an unhealthy society.

Thus, this book is meant for both men and women, and not for women only, despite its title.

२. स्त्री समाज की सबसे छोटी इकाई के बीज स्वरूप है तथा उसके असन्तोष से वर्तमान और भविष्य में संशय एवं अस्तव्यस्तता आ जाती है।

2. **Woman is the nucleus of the smallest social unit, and when she is not well, confusion and chaos prevail in the present and future.**

A woman is generally the central force of the family, since it is from her womb that the family proliferates. In pregnancy, child-birth, and breast-feeding she has an exclusive role. Her little ones depend upon her, cling to her breasts, and feel secure in her vicinity. A woman symbolizes earth, which provides protection, nourishment, and security. She is like a big banyan tree in whose cool shadow children and father find comfort. She is generous and abundant. This is her prakriti, her general nature, though of course there are exceptions. The intensity of motherhood depends upon the ratio of the male–female principle in each human being, a subject we'll discuss at length in later Parts of this book.

Woman's generosity does not mean, however, that others around her should take from her without due compensation. The relationship with a woman is like our relationship to earth. In ancient civilizations, the earth and its attributes—its rivers, lakes, mountains, trees, and vegetation—were worshipped. People showed their gratitude through ceremonies; in cases of natural catastrophe, they tried to appease its anger in various ways.

The people of modern industrial civilizations, however, have caused irreversible environmental blunders. After several centuries of exploitation, they have now become aware of the seriousness of their deeds and have begun attempts to heal the wounds. Some say that the roots of the exploitation of both nature and women were laid by the pioneers of modern science.[1] If those around a woman take undue advantage of her generosity, if they do not show their gratitude and respect for her, she becomes prey to discomfort and ailments, like mother earth.

This lack of well-being may influence the future. Ill health and the unhappy mental state of a woman adversely affect even her unborn children, who may themselves grow up to be insecure, frustrated mothers prone to mental problems. The happiness and health of a woman are important for our present and our future.

Talk of the well-being of women does not imply neglect of men and children. But if a woman is ignored and lives under conditions of mental pain and discomfort, children and their father will also suffer.

३. स्त्री को चाहिए कि वह संसार में शान्ति तथा सन्तुलन बनाने के लिए अपनी सुरक्षा का मार्ग तथा अपने हित का उपाय स्वयं ढूंढ़े।

3. A woman must learn to protect herself and take care of her own well-being, for the sake of cosmic harmony and balance.

A woman should protect herself and safeguard her own rights, rather than expect this from others. In her capacity as nucleus of the family, she can create better conditions for her own well-being and that of those around her.

First, her association with her male partner should be without confusion. She should not make him dependent upon her either emotionally or in household responsibilities. His dependence is good for neither of them. Some women make themselves indispensable to enhance their own sense of pleasure and pride, or to satisfy their egos, or to try to win the attention and love of their partners. In the process, they do great harm to themselves, though they realize it only much much later.

At the age they begin to cultivate such habits, they have plenty of energy. With the arrival of children and passing of time, responsibilities grow and stamina decreases. Dissatisfaction and irritation arise. A moment comes when they can no longer carry the load of their extensive responsibilities. This is why so many women suffer from physical and mental ailments in their mid-forties. At this stage in their lives, when they feel weak anyway because of the physiological changes taking place in their bodies, they often feel they "can't take it any longer," but find it nearly impossible to change the habits they have cultivated for so long.

Even a woman in a traditional patriarchal family structure who

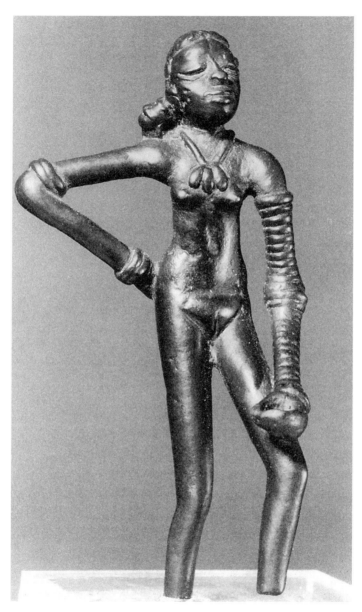

"Dancing Girl" from Mohenjodaro, ca. 3000 B.C.

does not work outside the house should not make her partner completely dependent upon her. In such a situation it is obvious she carries a bigger responsibility in the household, but she still needs leisure for herself. She should pursue hobbies and social work and not devote herself twenty-four hours a day to the family. Working outside the house makes others around her realize that she is not always there to help and serve them. If she does not, she is likely to suffer from many ailments, especially when her children leave the house and their father retires. A feeling of void may encircle her, giving rise to mental problems. With ill health and irritable behavior, she becomes a problem for everybody around her.

A woman may work for others out of generosity and love, but by making them dependent upon her for all the little things of life, she is only harming herself and them. It is pitiable when a grown man does not know where his clothes are, how to prepare a suitcase for traveling, how to organize food to nourish himself, or all the other small facts of life. If circumstances in life find such a man on his own, he feels completely lost and confused, and will often take almost anyone to fill his need.

Children brought up by mothers who do everything for them never become self-sufficient and self-assured. Their personalities do not develop properly, they never learn to decide for themselves, and they tend to grow up weak. Boys from such families may later become a burden upon their female partners. Girls may propagate further this negative tradition. The ultimate result is that everyone suffers, especially women.

A woman should not act as a mute servant for her family. She should make others realize in a subtle way their duties and responsibilities. This should be done in a slow and amicable manner. Crude, abrupt methods or a sudden change in behavior can provoke strong reaction and lead to an unpleasant atmosphere. A woman can work for her liberation in many subtle and diplomatic ways.

In many ancient societies, customs and rituals protected women. For example, in India, a woman lived in separate quarters during menstruation and did no household work. She was said to be "impure" during these three days, which isn't a very nice idea; but on its positive side, she had time to recuperate from the physical stress of menstruation and also had a few holidays from her routine work. There were similar ceremonies and codes of conduct for pregnant women. After childbirth, a woman did not work for forty days. This provided her time to regain her lost strength.

With the changing times, these old rituals are being lost. We must invent new rituals to protect and safeguard women's rights in the family. For example, those who cook regularly for their families should develop the custom that at least once a week, this responsibility is assumed by their male partners or grown-up children. During this time, the woman should stay away from the kitchen and not interfere. She should be served as others are served when she is doing the work. Many women are insecure about "their domain"—the kitchen—and do not like men to enter their territory. Some are convinced that when men enter the kitchen, they will make a mess. Even if they want their male partners to cook or help, they keep interfering and nagging.

Do not let your partners be single-tracked in life! Inspire them to learn the management of a kitchen! Food is life, and it is a pity to go on eating all your life like a blind person without having the sensuous experience of preparing food. In cooking, varied products of different color, form, taste, and smell mingle with each other, giving rise to a single and wholesome sensation. Cooking is not unlike a sexual experience. Do not deprive men of this pleasure. Try to be patient and indulgent when they enter the kitchen, and if you cannot, then at least try to keep aloof.

Women with jobs should not be cooking regularly in any event; in these situations the responsibilities of the household should be divided equally among the adults in the family. When a woman works eight hours a day outside the house and still runs the household, her youth withers fast and she becomes sexually passive. Many times, a man wonders why his partner has lost all the enthusiasm for sex she had before they lived together. He does not realize that after all her work, she simply has no physical energy left for sexual activity.

I have said much about men and children becoming dependent on women. But women should also share in those responsibilities which are often traditionally thought to be exclusively for men. Some examples: construction and renovation of a house, maintenance and repair of various household tools and appliances, and purchases of real estate, a car, furniture, and so on. Too often women show no interest in these activities and leave the entire responsibility to men.

A woman must also learn to protect herself at her place of work. The male colleagues of women in many different professions and many different countries expect them to perform tasks such as making coffee, keeping order and cleanliness in the office, and doing other such small jobs. I remember that in one of the research laboratories where I was working while abroad, the male technician took it for granted that his female colleague would clean the laboratory dishes.

The other side is that women themselves perpetrate such situations at work by resisting tasks they expect men to do. Instead, you should use your best efforts to learn your profession well, whatever it may be. A helpless person cannot be assertive and strong. Many women are convinced that they cannot handle machines or other jobs requiring mechanical knowledge. This is just a mental blockage. Such thoughts should never enter your mind—be open to new things!

Begin with full concentration of mind and a strong will, and you will certainly succeed. It is essential that women become self-sufficient and independent before becoming assertive.

४. अपनी शक्ति को बढ़ाने में ही स्त्री का हित है।

4. A woman's well-being lies in developing her inner strength.

Blaming society, parents, or one's culture for one's mental or physical weakness only leads to a bitter and grumbling attitude and does not bring any fruitful results. A woman who blames will spoil her mental state and acquire an unpleasant personality. Also, complaining about what is already done is only destructive. This does not mean a woman should not face the facts about her life. Rather, these facts should provide guidance, for herself and future generations. There is always time for a new beginning. Instead of dwelling upon what was, examine the debris, save what you can, then begin with a new foundation based on truth, kindness, humility, and generosity. The practical aspects of developing this strength are discussed throughout the book.

५. शक्ति तीन प्रकार की होती है : शारीरिक, मानसिक तथा आत्मिक।

5. Strength has physical, mental, and spiritual aspects.

The three types of strength just listed are in order of priority. Physical strength is the first essential, since without good health, you cannot easily find the means to pursue a livelihood. (In Ayurveda, it is said that the first priority of life is life itself; the second, to obtain the means of a livelihood, without which a long life can be miserable. It is only after fulfilling these two priorities that one should follow the path to spirituality.)[2]

Food, shelter, and clothing—the means of sustenance—are the primary human needs. After these needs are fulfilled, you can develop mental strength—itself a prerequisite for the spiritual path. Mind controls the mind, and it is only through the efforts of the mind that one can transcend physical reality.

६. शक्ति उसके अपने प्रयत्न से ही बढ़ेगी।

6. A woman develops strength through her own efforts.

All of us are born and brought up in different circumstances—some privileged, others having to strive hard just to get the simple things of life. According to the Hindu tradition, place and conditions of our birth depend upon the stock of our previous deeds, or *karma*. With our present karma (what we do now), we can bring our privileged condition to ruins or build a beautiful structure on the previous ruins. Therefore, the role of present karma, or personal effort, is very important.

७. प्रयत्न करना सबके लिए अनिवार्य है, उनके लिए भी जो जन्म से सौन्दर्ययुक्त तथा धनवान हैं।

7. Personal effort is essential in all cases, even for those born rich and beautiful.

Imagine someone born with good looks. In her youth, her beauty blooms. However, through careless behavior she gets fat, or through neglect she suffers from bad digestion and de-velops rough skin. Her beauty can also fade through irritable behavior. Through her present karma, she has lost what she had earned through her past karma. On the other hand, someone with moderate looks can make herself charming and attractive by taking care of her health and imbibing positive personality traits.

Without personal effort, a woman cannot develop the strength necessary for her well-being.

८. स्त्री की सच्ची सुन्दरता उसकी शक्ति में है, न कि उसके बाह्य रूप में ।

8. A woman's real beauty lies in her strength, not in her outward appearance.

This sutra should provide men with a good guideline for choosing their female partners. A charming outward appearance without inner strength, self-confidence, and ability to discern does not last long and is not a good base for sexual sharing. External physical beauty and sexuality are universally linked together, but when the mind lacks strength, one cannot have a fulfilling sexual experience.

We have discussed earlier the imbalance brought about when a man and children become dependent upon the woman. Here is the reverse example. A woman who lacks strength becomes a parasite on others around her. For a woman to lead an enriched, sexually fulfilling life, she must develop her strength, which will provide her with a radiant outlook (*tejas*) and make her attractive in every respect. To enhance the sensuous pleasure in sexuality requires sharpening the power of the senses. This can be done only with strong will power and persistence. A weak person gives up such efforts and cannot experience an intense sensual experience, though it is by intensifying the sensuous experience that one is able to prolong the experience of sexual bliss.

It has been observed that some women use elaborate makeup, color their hair, and adopt all sorts of other artificial means to attract the attention of a partner. Relationships which are based upon such artificial factors mostly end up in disaster. A woman who spends so much effort, time, and money on making herself attractive superficially is basically an unhappy person. Rather than seeking fulfillment through these artificial means, she should try to evoke a long-lasting beauty from within.

६. शारीरिक तथा मानसिक कोमलता और शक्ति समकालिक है।

9. Strength and flexibility of body and mind are acquired simultaneously.

Strength and flexibility of the body and mind can be acquired simultaneously through various yogic methods. As you know, yoga is not a mere physical exercise. The slow body movements in yoga are coordinated simultaneously with a concentration on breathing. The inhalation and exhalation of breath denotes our link to the cosmos. With a regular practice of yoga, both mind and body become relaxed. The body acquires flexibility, and the mind becomes peaceful. The concentration itself eventually leads to a thought-free mind.

In Part VI some specific yogic exercises are offered.

१०. चित्त के स्थिर होने से एकाग्रता होती है तथा एकाग्रता से आत्मज्ञान।

10. Stillness of the thinking process brings singlepointedness, which leads to spiritual lucidity.

When the mind is thought-free and still and this state is continuously maintained, the mind becomes one with the soul. Normally, the mind undergoes a continuous chain of thoughts and is connected to the world through the senses. The basic nature of the soul is still; it is free of qualities and changes. It is the cause of consciousness. However, when we acquire a thought-free mental state through personal efforts, the mind withdraws from sensuous experience and becomes one with the soul.

११. आत्मज्ञान से ही इन्द्रियों द्वारा काम की पूर्ण तृप्ति तथा आत्मा का साक्षात्कार होता है।

11. Spiritual lucidity is essential for attaining sensuous and spiritual fulfillment through sexuality.

This book does not deal exclusively with the sensuous experience of sex but also with the spiritual experience. To get spiritual experience from sexual union, you must develop the power of concentration that leads to stillness of the mind. Sensuous pleasure is enhanced by a flexible body and by the power of concentration and breathing practices.

All the five senses are involved in sexual interaction. With enhanced power of concentration, sensuality is taken to an utmost degree, a state where it actually ceases to be, and the mind attains stillness. This is the peak of the sexual experience. Extending this momentary stillness and having an experience of beatitude is the spiritual experience in sexuality, the moment when the thought-free mind withdraws from the senses and experiences oneness with the soul (see Part XI). A person who has already developed her or his power of concentration with *pranayama*—the yogic practices of breathing—can utilize this power for spiritual ends (see Part VII, Sutra 10).

नारी कामसूत्र के प्रथम भाग की यहां इति होती है। इसमें नारीत्व के बोध पर प्रकाश डाला गया है तथा पुस्तक के विषयों को संक्षेप में बताया गया है।

This brings to an end Part I of *The Kamasutra for Women* on self-awareness, introducing the theme of the book.

PART II
*H*armony in *M*ale and *F*emale *P*rinciples

· · ·

दूसरा भाग

स्त्री तत्व तथा पुरुष तत्व में सन्तुलन

· · ·

To enjoy the pleasures of *Kama*, the supreme universal energy
manifested itself in dual form. A black light (Krishana) impregnated
a white light (Radha).

—*Karapatri Svami*

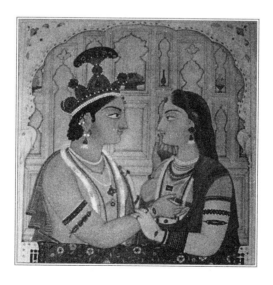

९. नर और नारी की मूल प्रकृति में अन्तर का कारण उनमें स्त्री तत्व के तथा पुरुष तत्व के अनुपात की भिन्नता है।

1. The basic natures of woman and man differ because of the difference in the ratio of female and male principles present in them.

There is always much discussion about this subject in all civilized societies. In many cultures, stereotypical characteristics are attributed to one or the other sex, damaging the tenderness and flexibility of nearly all relationships. Men are trained to be unyielding, adamantine, unstirred by any emotion. Being so hard to themselves, holding back their emotions, they develop ailments such as stomach ulcers, piles, colitis, and so on.

Women, on the other hand, are taught to become only mothers and wives, to serve and care. They are shielded from the tough activities of life and made to feel completely helpless if they have to face the external world. In ancient cultures and in tribal societies, such compartmentalization was/is not made, and the profoundness of the separation and union of two sexes was/is better understood than in modern, technologically advanced societies.

Masculine and feminine principles exist within both man and woman, but the ratio varies in each—as well as within the same sex. Expressions such as "a feminine man" or "a masculine woman" are very common in many languages and are used to describe individuals in whom this ratio is thought to be too lopsided.

I will try to express this idea in a mathematical way, for the sake of clarity. Let us suppose that according to the norms of a particular society, a perfect woman has 80 percent of the female and 20 percent of the male principle. She may be designated as being "very feminine." The percentages vary and help account for a wide range of characteristics. Let us suppose most women come with a masculine principle in the range between 21 percent to 35 percent.

Perhaps, above 35 percent a woman shows characteristics which strike others as being strongly masculine, and she is therefore designated a "masculine woman." We can apply the same numerical example to describe a "feminine man."

Remember, however, that these numerical examples are only illustrations to help explain the sutra; these principles cannot really be thought about in terms of numbers, which have no validity as such. Using this terminology of male and female principles signifies a form of energy or force rather than something concrete. It should also be understood that in these examples, the male–female principles do not refer only to external masculine and feminine qualities but represent the inherent characteristics and innate qualities of both sexes.

२. स्त्री तत्व तथा पुरुष तत्व त्रिगुणात्मक हैं तथा तीनों गुणों की मात्रा में भिन्नता उनके भेद का कारण है।

2. Three fundamental qualities make up the female and male principles; it is the ratio of these qualities that makes them different from each other.

The three fundamental qualities mentioned in this sutra are *sattva, rajas,* and *tamas.* These are the three basic qualities of the Cosmic Substance, the Prakriti. The union of the Universal Soul, the Purusha, and the Cosmic Substance, the Prakriti, is the cause of the phenomenal world. The Purusha is without any substance and qualities. It is the energy, the animating principle of the Prakriti. (See the following box for details.)

Sattva is the quality of truth, beauty, goodness, virtue, and equilibrium. Rajas is the quality that denotes force, impetus, and action. Tamas restrains, restricts, obstructs, and resists motion. Sattva is the quality of light and knowledge; rajas, of motion and action; and tamas, of darkness and inaction. These three qualities are interrelated and influence each other, like the three sides of a triangle; when one side changes, it affects the other two.

To keep a balance in the three qualities is more difficult then to maintain an equilibrium in pairs of opposite qualities.[1] The three qualities should not be confused with the Yin and Yang of the Chinese tradition, which refer to two opposite poles of energy. Everything in the phenomenal world has these three qualities in variable ratio. The three qualities form the entire nature of the universe at various subtle and practical levels of our existence and are also applied to other cosmic phenomena.

Sattva is an individual's cause of existence; it denotes soul. It can be compared to the state of wakefulness. (The terms *sleep*, *dream*, and *wakefulness* are used in an abstract manner here.) The soul is the cause of being of the material body. Thus, it is the real "Self" of an individual.

Tamas is often compared to the state of sleep. An embryo is in a state of tamas before it is born.

Rajas is often compared to a state of dream. It denotes the activities of life which take place with the inner subtle energy.

In relation to the body, the tamas, rajas, and sattva represent the physical, the subtle, and the spiritual aspects of human existence.

From a cosmic view, tamas is the devouring principle of the universe, rajas is the creative principle, and sattva is the principle of energy and life.

There is more sattva and tamas than rajas in the female principle. In the male principle, rajas dominates, while sattva and tamas are lesser. It is the ratio of these qualities that makes the male and female principles different from each other.

In modern technologically advanced civilizations, with their hectic pace of life, lack of real leisure, and lack of time for spiritual pursuits, all three qualities are in a state of imbalance, giving rise to many problems that play themselves out in the relationships between men and women, including sexuality.

THE PHILOSOPHICAL BASIS
OF YOGA AND AYURVEDA

The combination of the two fundamental forces is responsible for the phenomenal world. These are the Purusha (or Universal Soul) and the Prakriti (or Cosmic Substance). Let us call the Purusha A and the Prakriti B. A is the animating principle of B. A is without qualities or substance; it is that which breathes life into B. The Prakriti has three constituent qualities, which are called *sattva* (quality of truth, virtue, beauty, and equilibrium), *rajas* (quality of force and impetus), and *tamas* (quality that restrains, restricts, and hinders motion). Despite these qualities, the Prakriti does not have any urge to act, as it is inanimate. Only with the combination of A and B does existence manifest itself.

The combination of A and B leads to the existence of three principal factors: intellect or power of discretion, individuating principle, and power of thinking or mind. These three give rise to five subtle elements: sound, touch, appearance, flavor, and odor. With these elements, the universe becomes a reality vis-à-vis "me" (individuating principle), as it is through these subtle elements that "I" am able to perceive the universe made of five fundamental elements.

The fundamental elements are ether, air, fire (or light), water, and earth. The whole universe is made of these five elements. Related to the five subtle elements are the five senses: hearing, feeling, sight, taste, and smell. The senses operate through their respective fundamental elements. For example, the medium for the sense of hearing is sound, which operates through ether. Related to the five senses are the five modes of action: the capacity to express, grasp, move, excrete, and procreate (Table 1).

Before the combination of the Universal Soul and the Cosmic Substance, the three qualities are in a state of perfect balance. After the combination, the balance of the three qualities changes constantly, due to actions, or karma. The karma is the inherent nature of the phenomenal world.

The universe is a constantly changing dynamic whole, where

everything is interconnected, interrelated, and interdependent. There is constant transformation, and this transformation denotes time. Birth, death, and the different stages of life are nothing but transformations from one state to another. Nothing is ever lost, and nothing happens without a reason. Everything moves towards a definite goal.

Our body is constituted of the five basic elements. However, the cause of consciousness is the soul, a part of the Universal Soul. The soul, itself without any substance or qualities, is the animating principle. When the soul leaves the body, a person is dead. The body degenerates and the five elements, which were in a specific bodily organization, return to their main pool. The soul, or *jiva*, acquires a new body in the womb of the mother and is said to be reborn.

The conditions and circumstances of birth depend upon the individual's karma. In this way, we undergo a constant cycle of life and death, called *sansara*. The cycle of birth and death is painful because of the quality of impermanence. All we love and accumulate, we have to leave. Nothing is permanent. Liberation lies in seeking the path of immortality and getting rid of the cycle of birth and death forever. We do this by recognizing our real self—the soul—as distinguished from the body. The soul is immortal and permanent.

Yoga teaches the techniques of attaining mastery over one's senses and reaching the realm of soul. The aim of Yoga is to attain the complete separation of soul from the body. But due to previous karma, it is not possible to liberate the soul from the body, as the remains of karma, called *sanskara*, remain with each individual soul, which drag it from womb to womb. One gets rid of sanskara only through *samadhi*, the last of the three stages of mind after attaining a thought-free state.[2]

Table 1   A Summary of the Speculation on Cosmic Reality
According To the Concepts of the *Sankhya* and Yoga

Animating principle of B. It is without any qualities or substance and thus cannot act alone.	+	Has three fundamental qualities. It has substance but cannot act alone, as it is inanimate.

All existence manifests itself when A breathes life into B.
This combination gives rise to

↓

Power of discretion + Individuating principle + Mind

These three make the world real vis-à-vis "me"
through five subtle elements, which are

↓

Sound + Touch + Appearance + Flavor + Odor

It is through these subtle elements that one becomes capable
of perceiving the universe made of the five basic elements,
which are

↓

Ether + Air + Fire + Water + Earth

The combination of all these gives rise to five sense organs
and five modes of action, which are

↓

**Hearing + Feeling + Seeing + Tasting + Smelling
+   +   +   +   +
Expressing + Grasping + Moving + Excreting + Procreating**

३. स्त्री तत्व तथा पुरुष तत्व के अनुपात में भिन्नता के कारण स्त्री
और पुरुष की मूल प्रकृति में अन्तर होता है।

3. The difference in the ratio of the male and female principles in men and women is the cause for the difference in the inherent nature of the two sexes.

Let us try to understand this with the same kind of mathematical ratios we used to explain Sutra 1. Suppose that the male principle is defined in the abstract as consisting of 50 percent rajas and 25 percent each of tamas and sattva, while the female principle consists of 40 percent each sattva and tamas and just 20 percent rajas. A woman with 20 percent of the male principle and 80 percent of the female principle will contain 26 percent rajas and 37 percent of sattva and of tamas. A man with 80 percent of male principle and 20 percent of female principle will have 44 percent rajas and 28 percent of tamas and of sattva. The variations in ratio are basically infinite and can help explain the differences in people's sexual expression and behavior. As has been said earlier, these numbers are mere suppositions for the facility of understanding. They have no validity as such.

The innate attributes of women and men emerge from the different ratios of the three qualities. The male attributes involve activity, action, and movement. The female attributes are stillness, spirituality, creation, nursing, and so on. These characteristics can be readily observed in young children. Little girls are usually more peaceful, stable, and calm than little boys, who jump and move a great deal. Girls often play with dolls, taking care of them, nursing them, and putting them to sleep. Some say these characteristics are the result of the imposition of social norms by the parents. It is not true. If it were, all the mothers who are exhausted by the mischievous behavior of their little boys would be able to manipulate them easily.

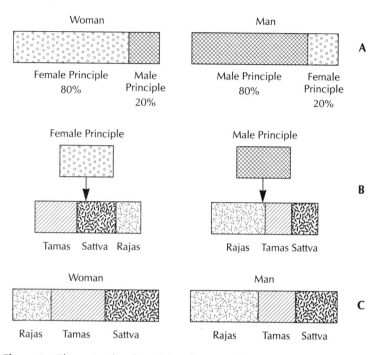

Figure 1   The ratio of male and female principles in a man and a woman (see Sutras 1–3) are represented. *A* shows a hypothetical example of a woman and a man with a female and male ratio of 80%:20% and 20%:80%, respectively. *B* shows that both male and female principles have three fundamental qualities of nature—sattva, rajas, and tamas (represented by different designs in the figure)—but in different ratios. The female principle is hypothetically shown to contain 26% of rajas and 37% of tamas and of sattva. The male principle contains 44% of rajas and 28% of sattva and of tamas. *C* represents a woman and man with varying ratio of the three qualities interpreted in terms of hypothetical percentages shown in *A* and *B*.

• • •

Figure 1 shows a diagrammatic representation of the ideas expressed in the above three sutras.

४. मातृत्व स्त्रीत्व का एक अभिन्न अंग है तथा वह केवल सन्तान उत्पत्ति से सम्बन्ध नहीं रखता।

4. Motherhood is an innate feminine quality, related not only to having a child.

As used here, the word *feminine* does not mean "women." Feminine or masculine exist in differing proportions in both men and women, and both feminine and masculine attributes are very diverse.

The innate quality of motherhood is attributed generally only to women, and that, too, is associated mostly with childbirth. Yet motherhood exists in all of us in varying degrees: it is the quality of providing protection and care, of expressing tenderness and affection. It is a sattvic quality, the quality of *karuna*, or compassion. Due to the difference in ratio in the three fundamental qualities, women have it in abundance, men less so. In some societies, this quality is suppressed in men. Without any regard to the variation in individual character and with no respect for the ratio of masculine and feminine principles, men are pushed to take on such roles as soldier, surgeon, hunter, or medical researcher. Those men who have more of a quality of motherhood than others suffer greatly, and they may get ill.

A free expression of the basic human quality of motherhood should be allowed for the health of men and women and society. It exists within us not only to help us rear children but also to play an important role in sexuality. It is the responsibility of a woman to encourage the expression of this quality in the men around her and not to impose false values upon her little boys.

५. स्त्रियों की स्वाधीनता तथा स्वतन्त्रता एवं पुरुषों का प्रभुत्व अपने अन्दर के मातृत्व भाव को अस्वीकार करने में नहीं होता।

5. The liberation and freedom of women and the supremacy of men do not lie in denying the inherent element of motherhood in either of them.

In some societies, men and women are compartmentalized and assigned different duties. In the process, women get too engrossed in household activities, and men get excessively involved in life outside their homes. Men become remote from their families and women, overly attached. Equilibrium in society is lost. Both men and women are denying some of their innate natural qualities, and imbalances arise over a period of time. Women are prone to depression, or they acquire an irritable and angry character due to an excess of tamas. Tamas may also cause an accumulation of *kapha*, one of the three body humors, in some parts of their bodies, blocking the flow of energy and creating disease. I will go into detail about the humors in Sutra 2 of Part III.

The well-being of men, women, and the society lies in our not suppressing our innate qualities and denying a part of our being. If men are taught to become hard and tough and to deny the expression of tenderness which is a natural inborn character in all of them, if they are denied such natural privileges as holding a baby, they are denied a free outlet of their emotions. The degree of the problem depends upon the ratio of female principle in a particular man.

Men with a relatively higher percentage of feminine principle undergo considerable emotional damage in societies where a constant force is exerted upon them to be masculine. Their behavior does not fit in with the attributes expected of a male regardless of natural variations. In denying their basic nature to fulfill the expectations of women and society, some men take recourse in a lonely life or homosexuality.

It is essential to recognize the presence of different degrees of the feminine principle in men. A woman should encourage her male partner to participate in those activities where he can express his innate quality of motherhood, including child rearing. Existing norms that encourage the segregation of men and women should be ignored. Women should proceed with wisdom, understanding, and patience and should bring up their male children by teaching them about the fundamental variety and flexibility of

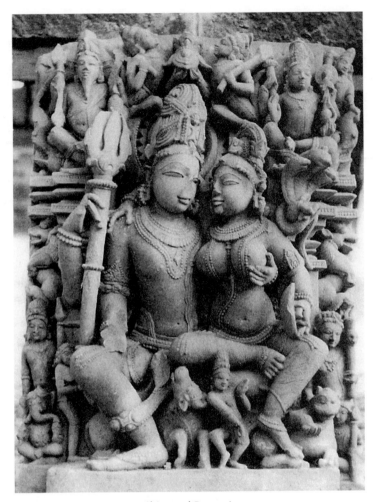

Shiva and Paravati.

human beings. Women also suffer from ignorance about the variations in male–female principles and characteristics. The roles of mother and wife are often imposed upon them, in denial of other needs. This imposition has finally given rise to a reactionary uprising that has asserted the false ideology that, for women, freedom and liberation lie in denying the expression of their mother-hood. Women who subscribe to this ideology feel that in order to be liberated, they have to be like men. Instead of encouraging men to become more flexible and tender, such reactionary women try to be hard and tough, and they deny themselves children and the beauty of being tender, compassionate, and expressive in their emotions. This does not lead to freedom. Real freedom lies in developing physical, mental, and spiritual strength. The denial of the innate strong quality of motherhood contravenes the principles of nature and a woman's own self.

Liberation and freedom of women are more subtle than this. To heal the wounds caused to the eternal mother (i.e., the mother earth and the feminine principle), we need to work together with men. The feminine principle within them has also suffered. The reactionary attitude of women in the recent past has increased the sufferings of men, not to mention children. Ironically, some women go on fighting with grown men (father, brother, husband, etc.) all their lives for their rights, and they do nothing to influence their own male children on this subject.

६. सृष्टि के त्रिगुणात्मक होने के कारण गुणों का अनुपात सदैव बदलता रहता है।

6. The three fundamental qualities are also present in the whole cosmos, and their ratio is constantly changing.

The universe is an ever-changing, dynamic whole, where nothing is static and everything is interdependent, interrelated, and interconnected. This constant change in the phenomenal world is the result of constant change in the three fundamental qualities, change that comes about through action, or karma. Our present karma (what we do now) can alter the ratio of these basic qualities, which are present in all cosmic phenomena. What we eat, how we live, how we sleep, how we behave—all these influence the qualities. If we eat a particular food which is dominant in certain qualities, it will affect our thinking process and hence our actions.

This is why a yoga adept should eat only sattvic food, such as rice, milk, ghee, carrots, and zucchini. Persons seeking worldly pleasures and sensuous joy should eat rajasic food, which include varieties of fruits and vegetables, cheese, some easy-to-digest meats, and foods prepared in the "right" combinations. Tamasic food is sleep inducing and inhibits action. Hard-to-digest and strong-smelling foods, such as onions and pork, belong in this category.

For equilibrium and harmony, a worldly person should eat food balanced with respect to the three fundamental qualities. These three varieties of food affect the body's three humors. (The sattvic, rajasic, and tamasic affect pitta, vata, and kapha, respectively; again, these humors are explained early in the next chapter.) The variation in the ratio of these qualities particularly hits women over the course of their lifetimes because of such physiological changes as menstruation, pregnancy, childbirth, and menopause. It is important to try always to maintain harmony of the three qualities. (The reader should understand that many food products combine several qualities and cannot be strictly categorized. For example, garlic is tamasic, but in small quantities in appropriate combination, also rajasic.)

७. मनुष्य को अपना पूरा मनोबल तथा अपनी बुद्धि तीनों गुणों का सन्तुलन बनाये रखने के लिए लगानी चाहिए।

7. Human willpower and discretion should be used to seek an equilibrium among the three qualities.

For example, when you have a tamas-dominated period (as is the case a few days before menstruation), you should make an effort to get out of the darkness and gloom by wearing bright clothes, by eating rajasic food, and by exercising willpower. You need to observe very carefully the quality of your actions and their effect, and use your power of discretion to undertake actions that compensate for the lack of one quality or the excess of the other.

८. सृष्टि के सन्तुलन के लिए यह आवश्यक है कि स्त्री और पुरुष अपने को एक दूसरे के पूरक समझे न कि अलग अलग खण्ड।

8. For cosmic harmony, both women and men should realize their oneness and not remain in segregated compartments.

Every woman has a man in her and every man, a woman in him. They are both within each other. Together, they complete each other, and their union leads to cosmic harmony. Segregation and compartmentalization result in clashes of values, as well as confusion in sharing responsibility and exercising authority. Comprehending the oneness of man and woman can lead to more flexibility in the relationship and more patience for one another. Instead of denying the other certain desires or privileges, we should search out those needs within ourselves to better understand the other.

Let us take some examples. After childbirth, a woman gets very much involved with her baby. Actually, she has already been with the baby during the nine months of pregnancy. Even if she is a professional woman, her activities are already focused on the formation and well-being of her child. Sooner or later comes a natural balance in her professional and motherly activities.

However, the arrival of the baby often gives the father a feeling of deprivation, especially if he suppresses the quality of motherhood within himself and does not make an effort to develop a relationship with his baby. Many men think that their relationship with their child begins only later when he or she begins to go to school. This is a false idea. Nine months of pregnancy are the exclusive privilege of a woman, but immediately after the beginning of motherhood, care and protection should be provided by both parents.

Duties and relationships are two different things. Fulfilling material needs is perhaps the duty of the father in certain cases. But the expression of his motherhood builds up his relationship with the baby and provides him relief from his dominant rajas quality. Even if he is tired, working for his baby will provide him more energy and will invigorate him, due to the balance in qualities. His sexual relationship with the mother of his child will also rejuvenate. The woman, on her part, should generously and wisely share her motherhood with her partner. If she becomes possessive about the child and thinks that she is the only one who can take care of her or him, she too may suffer.

Certain notions about the division of duties between men and women that were perhaps necessary a century ago have no more validity in our modern, technologically advanced societies. These old values can become a hindrance today. In former times, a lot of labor was required to keep a household and bring up children; it was not possible for middle-class women to pursue a profession while performing their duties as mothers and wives. Men's professions were also tougher and required more time and energy. Technological and psychological evolutions have not gone hand in hand, however; a housewife today seldom feels "indispensable" as she once did. If she becomes frustrated and feels unfulfilled, this may destroy family harmony. With the wide availability of restaurants and the "food revolution," men are also less reliant on women's "making the home." In former times the marital bond was not easily broken because a couple could not afford to break it. The validity of this statement is proved when we observe that high rates of divorce exist only in affluent, technologically advanced societies, where the basic material need to stay together no longer exists.

With the changing times and needs, it is more essential than ever to work on the subtle psychological levels of male–female relationship and to rid ourselves of the idea of the segregation of men and women. It is not easy to bring social changes, and doing so will require time and tremendous effort at all levels by both men and women.

९. पुरुष अपने में पहले से अधिक गुण को और बढ़ाये तो उसमें रजोगुण का अंश अत्याधिक हो जाता है जो कि उसे स्त्री और बच्चों से दूर कर रोगों का कारण बनता है।

9. **Emphasis of man on his dominant quality results in too much rajas, an imbalance which makes him remote from his companion and children and leads to ailments.**

Some men are convinced that their role as men is fulfilled only when they are extremely successful in their careers. As already said, rajas dominates the male principle. With a desire to get ahead, some men get too involved in their profession. Overactivity, excessive work, and too much interaction with other people further amplifies rajas. Such men do not have time to sit and relax, play with their children, or just have quiet moments. Excess of rajas may lead to insomnia, restlessness, nervous disorders, hypertension, and so on. This overactivity involves a suppression of the female principle within him, creating an imbalance with serious consequences. A man should take care not to let his rajas overcome him, and he should make it a point to spend time with children or friends or participate in social events and ceremonies. He should devote a part of his time every day to breathing and concentration exercises.

१०. अगर स्त्री ऐसा करे तो उसका भी यही दुष्परिणाम होता है।

10. **A woman meets a similar fate if she emphasizes her already dominant qualities.**

As noted earlier, a woman has more tamas and sattva in her than rajas. It is the dominant tamas quality which gives a woman the desire to make a home and to be in one place. A combination of rajas and tamas leads to the desire to have a family. Sattva gives rise to qualities like goodness, generosity, compassion, kindness, devotion, and the search for inner peace and stillness. Due to the dominance of sattva in women, you will find that in yoga-meditation groups and other spiritual pursuits, there is a larger percentage of women. Credit for preserving the ancient tradition of India goes largely to women.

Some women, however, get too involved in spiritual pursuits and ignore the material part of life, disturbing familial harmony. There are other women who emphasize their tamas quality by staying too much indoors and sleeping excessively. This may lead to obesity, depression, and other such disorders. Women who do not work outside the house should pay particular attention here. Women as a rule have less rajas than men, and they should not try to suppress this quality. Women need to cultivate the activity of both body and mind.

Some women who react to an unhappy existence as a housewife suddenly want to take up a profession and begin an active outdoor life. If done too suddenly, this change can give rise to excessive rajas and have the same results as described for men in the previous sutra. Every effort should be made to keep the three fundamental qualities in equilibrium. Extreme reactions should be avoided. Women should act positively rather than reacting.

११. स्त्री पुरुष में कामपूर्ति एवं सहचरता के लिये गुणों को स्वतन्त्र रूप में प्रकट करना तथा एक दूसरे के गुणों के लिये सद्भाव रखना अनिवार्य है।

11. Free expression and understanding of each other's qualities are essential for sexual fulfillment and companionship between woman and man.

Only with understanding, patience, and generosity for each other can men and women lead a harmonious existence. For example, a woman should not be excessively assertive but should

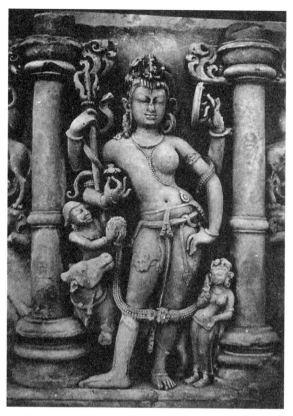

Aradhanarishvara, the symbol of Shiva and Shakti, of male-female union. The figure is half man and half woman, hence the one breast.

let the man express his rajas quality by participating in events that involve action and movement. If his expression of rajas is excessive, she should keep control on it in a subtle way by involving him in practices that bring stillness to the mind. For his part, a man should understand a woman's desire for family and home, yet encourage, not suppress, her rajas. He should get her involved in activities outside the home. If the rajas in her is suppressed, tamas increases, leading to anguish, depression, and sometimes outbursts of anger. He should also understand her gentle quality of motherhood and not be angry at her for being indulgent with her children.

नारी कामसूत्र के दूसरे भाग की यहां इति होती है। इसमें
स्त्री तत्व तथा पुरुष तत्व के त्रिगुणात्मक स्वरूप
के बारे में बताया गया है।

This brings to an end Part II of *The Kamasutra for Women*, describing the male female principles and the fundamental qualities that cause them.

PART III

Menstruation and Sexuality

. . .

तीसरा भाग

आर्तव का काम से सम्बन्ध

. . .

Bronze gets cleaned with acid,
river gets cleaned by its own forceful flow,
and a woman is purified with menstruation.
—*Canakya*

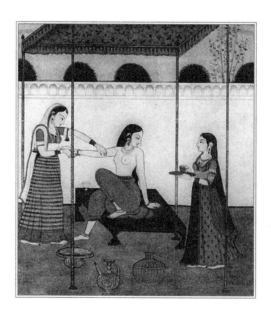

१. अपने जीवन को सुचारु रूप से चलाने के लिए स्त्री को मासिक
   धर्म के कारणों तथा प्रक्रिया के विषय में वैज्ञानिक जानकारी प्राप्त
   करनी चाहिए।

   **1. A woman should understand the exact process and cause
   of menstruation in order to better understand herself and
   gain a grip on her own life.**

A woman's sexual maturity, usually attained between twelve
to fourteen years of age, is marked by the release of blood for
three to five days every month. The two ovaries are located in
the lower part of the abdomen and measure approximately 1 inch
to 1 2/3 inches in length, about 1/2 half to 1 inch in width, and
about 1/4 to 1/2 of an inch in thickness (2.5 to 4 cm long, 1.2 to
2.5 cm wide, and .6 to 1.2 cm thick). The formation of the eggs
takes place in the ovaries. Both ovaries are connected to the
uterus by the oviducts, or fallopian tubes, which provide the egg
an appropriate environment for its fertilization and passage to the
uterus.

The uterus is a pear-shaped organ with a cavity inside and a
thick, muscular wall. In nonpregnant condition, it is about 2 inches
long, 1 inch wide, and 5/6 of an inch thick (5 cm long, 2.5 cm wide,
and 2 cm thick). In a sexually mature female, an egg is released
every month from one of her ovaries and descends to the uterus
through one of the fallopian tubes. The cavity of the uterus provides shelter to the fertilized egg, which transplants itself on its wall
and begins to grow into an embryo. Figure 2 shows a schematic
diagram of the female reproductive organs.

The inner lining of the wall of the uterus (facing the uterine
cavity) is called the endometrium. The endometrium prepares
itself every month for a fertilized egg. Its cells multiply and prepare a cushiony layer, but in the absence of fertilization, this layer
is sloughed off at the end of a four-week cycle. The cyclic changes
in the endometrium are controlled by the hormones estrogen and

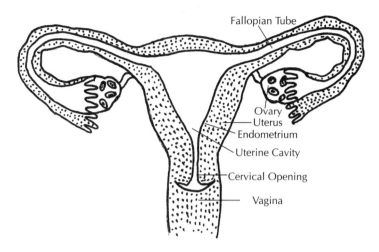

Fallopian Tube

Ovary
Uterus
Endometrium
Uterine Cavity

Cervical Opening

Vagina

Figure 2   The female reproductive organs.

progesterone, which are released in different parts of the body. These changes can be divided into two phases. After menstruation, a proliferative phase between day 5 to 14 begins under the influence of estrogen. The endometrium grows about .04 to .20 inches during this phase. From day 15 to 28 comes the secretory phase, so called because of the formation and secretion of glycogen. Glycogen is the cellular storehouse of sugar. The secretory phase is preceded by the synthesis of estrogen and progesterone, during which the endometrium increases by .12 to .31 inches. All this is a part of the necessary preparation for the transplantation of the fertilized egg.

Towards the last part of the secretory phase, an accumulation of extracellular fluid and an increased amount of mucus cause the endometrial cells to become progressively looser. The hyperhydrated cells retain plenty of water during this last stage, while a constriction of the arteries reduces the blood flow, leading to the degeneration of a part of the endometrium. The constricted arteries rupture, there is a hemorrhage, and a part of the endometrial layer is shed. From the remaining basal layer of the endometrium, regeneration takes place again and the next cycle begins.

This is a brief description of the process and cause of menstruation. It is important to understand that the changes occurring in the endometrium are not merely some localized physiological changes. They are caused by hormones. The release of hormones takes place elsewhere in the body, and their alteration affects the whole of the body processes.

२. मासिक धर्म की अवधि में स्त्री में शारीरिक तथा मानसिक परिवर्तन होते हैं ; अपना सन्तुलन बनाये रखने के लिए उसे पूरा प्रयत्न करना चाहिए।

2. A woman undergoes mental and physical changes during the period of the cycle, and she should make every effort to maintain equilibrium and harmony.

The various periods of the menstrual cycle are dominated by different humors, and it is important to understand them well to maintain equilibrium. Before we proceed, it is necessary to give a further introduction to the theory of five elements and the body humors.

According to the Ayurvedic principles of health, the body is constituted of five fundamental elements—ether, air, fire, water, and earth. These in turn give rise to the three bodily humors—*vata*, *pitta*, and *kapha*. These humors govern all physical and mental functions of the body. Where sattva, rajas, and tamas exist as abstract *qualities*, these three are the three vital *forces*, and they exist on the bodily plane. An equilibrium of the humors is essential to maintain the body in good health, vitality, and resistance to maladies.

Since everything in this universe has humoral qualities, the humors are constantly affected. For good health and harmony, a woman must live according to her own constitution, time, and place. Health should be the first priority, as without it, neither the worldly pleasures nor the spiritual experience leading to liberation is possible.

THE THREE HUMORS

Vata is constituted by the elements ether and air, and it is responsible for entire body movements and mind activities—that is, blood circulation, respiration, excretion, speech, sensation, touch, hearing, natural urges, formation of the foetus, the sexual act, retention, and feelings like fear, anxiety, grief, and enthusiasm. An excess of rajas, especially among men, may hamper the vata, impeding the body functions and giving rise to such diseases as hypertension, nervousness, and sleep-related disorders.

Pitta comes from fire and is responsible for vision, digestion, hunger, thirst, heat regulation, softness and luster, cheerfulness, intellect and sexual vigor.

Kapha comes from the basic elements earth and water, and it constitutes all the solid structure of the body. It is responsible for unctuousness, binding, firmness, heaviness, sexual potency, strength, forbearance, and restraint.

The three humors go on altering constantly in this ever-changing universe. They are interdependent and interrelated. The vitiation of one humor affects the others, and if not attended to, all the humors slowly vitiate. For example, excess of vata dries up kapha in the body. Vata is from ether and air, and like these two elements, it is mobile and all pervasive. One of the constituting elements of kapha is water. The wind always dries up water. A person with vitiated vata will often have dry skin or dry throat, because the excess of vata hinders the excretory functions of the cells, which is the domain of kapha.

On the other hand, excess of kapha hinders the free flow of vata and thus the distribution of energy in different parts of the body. Excess of pitta produces more latent heat in the body and diminishes kapha. Excess of kapha subdues the bodily fire (pitta) because water and earth can extinguish fire. Similarly, excess of vata causes an uneven distribution of pitta and vitiates it.

It is easy to understand the concept of humors by thinking of the functions of the five elements in the universe. Wind is a life-giving force, and we cannot survive without it. But excess of wind causes catastrophes, uprooting trees, destroying buildings, downing power lines, and disrupting all activities of life. A life-giving river becomes lethal when it drowns villages and fields during a flood.

The three humors of our body are made of these five elements, and the humors are the life-giving force when in equilibrium. However, when the humors lose their balance, they cause catastrophes in the body. Disorders due to the imbalance of humors are called innate disorders. Some examples of this category are hypertension, diabetes, various digestive problems, hemorrhoids, colitis, and sleep disorders. The imbalance of humors also brings down the *ojas* (immune response and vitality) of the body, making one prone to diseases.

In the context of sexuality, the three humors have different roles which help to coordinate the various sexual functions. If the humors are not in equilibrium, it is not possible to obtain a blissful sexual experience. Vata is responsible for sexual capacity. It is not possible to prolong sexual activity if this humor is vitiated. Pitta is responsible for sexual vigor. Vitiation of this humor will cause lack of intensity of sexual experience and sexual energy. Kapha is responsible for sexual excretions, and its lack may diminish sexual pleasure and cause infertility.

==== HOW TO DETERMINE YOUR ====
CONSTITUTION THROUGH
THE HUMOR TABLES

Learning to determine your constitution with the help of the humor tables given here is an essential tool in maintaining inner balance. Observe yourself carefully and make a list of the dominating traits you possess. (If the information given here is not sufficient to determine your constitution, refer to my other works on the subject, where you'll find other diagnostic methods.) After you have determined your basic constitution, take all necessary measures to forestall further enhancement of your dominating humor, to maintain equilibrium, and to eat according to place, time, and your individual need (Fig. 3 and Tables 2–7).[1] Do not necessarily adopt or reject foods globally described as healthy or unhealthy: something which may be very good for someone else may harm you because of your different constitution. For example, garlic is very good for general health and helps to increase immunity, but if you are a pitta-dominated person, you must take it in moderate quantities. If your pitta is vitiated, do not take garlic until you have reestablished your lost equilibrium.

Please understand that vitiation of a humor is not simply its excess. Vitiation may be caused due to an accumulation of a humor at a certain place, obviously causing "excess" at that particular place. Or else, a humor may be at the wrong place at a wrong time. For example, one of the functions of kapha is the formation of new cells to replace the old, including the formation of secretory cells. The formation of cells at an undesired place is pathological and is also termed "vitiation" of kapha.

Pitta is responsible for digestion and assimilation of the various digestive juices that act upon the food. However, the secretion of these juices without the presence of food to be digested is pathological and is also termed "vitiation."

Table 2   Origin, Functions, and Characteristics of Vata

Vata is light, subtle, mobile, dry, cold, rough, and all pervasive like the basic elements (air and ether) it is derived from.

Vata is responsible for entire body movements and mind activities, blood circulation, respiration, excretion, speech, sensation, touch, hearing, feelings like fear, anxiety, grief, and enthusiasm, natural urges, formation of the foetus, the sexual act, and retention.

Vata-Dominated People	Factors that Increase Vata	Signs of Vitiated Vata	Treatment of Vitiated Vata
• agile	• fasting	• general stiffness and pain in the body	• sweet, sour, and hot therapeutic measures
• quick and unrestricted in their movements	• excessive physical exercise	• bad taste and dryness in the mouth	• enema
• swift in action	• exposure to cold	• lack of appetite	• vata-decreasing diet
• quick in fear and other emotions	• laziness	• stomachache	• massage
• get easily irritated	• keeping awake late at night	• dry skin	• anointing
• intolerant to cold and shiver easily	• rainy season	• fatigue	• appropriate rest, relaxation, and sleep
• have coarse hairs and nails	• old age	• dark stools	• peaceful atmosphere
• have prominent blood vessels	• evening and last part of the night	• insomnia	• cheerful mental state
	• eating overripe and dry food and food that is kept a long time after cooking	• pain in temporal region	
	• injury	• giddiness	
	• blood loss	• tremors	
	• excessive sexual intercourse	• yawning	
	• anxiety	• hiccups	
	• uneven posture	• malaise	
	• suppression of natural urges	• delirium	
	• guilt	• dull complexion	
		• withdrawn and timid behavior	

From *Ayurveda: A Way of Life* by Vinod Verma

Table 3   Origin, Functions, and Characteristics of Pitta

Pitta is hot like the basic element fire it is derived from. It is also characteristic in being sharp, sour, and pungent, with a fleshy smell.

Pitta is responsible for vision, digestion, hunger, thirst, heat regulation, softness and luster, cheerfulness, intellect, and sexual vigor.

Pitta-Dominated People	Factors that Increase Pitta	Signs of Vitiated Pitta	Treatment of Vitiated Pitta
• intolerant to heat	• sharp, alkaline, salty foods	• excessive perspiration	• sweet, bitter, astringent, cold measures
• usually have hot face	• any food or drink which creates a burning sensation	• smell in the body	• unction and purgation
• delicate organs	• sun bathing	• abnormal hunger and thirst	• fasting
• tendency to have moles, freckles, pimples (acne)	• noontime	• inflammation	• cold bath and massage
• lustrous complexion	• midnight	• tearing and thickening of skin	• special pitta-decreasing diet
• excessive hunger and thirst	• autumn	• rash	• consolation
• early appearance of wrinkles	• process of digestion	• acne	
• falling and graying hairs	• youth	• herpes	
• body smell	• anger	• excessive heat in the body	
• intolerance and lack of endurance		• burning sensation	
		• loss of contentment	
		• dissatisfaction	
		• anger	

From *Ayurveda: A Way of Life* by Vinod Verma

Table 4   Origin, Functions, and Characteristics of Kapha

Kapha is derived from the basic elements earth and water. Like these elements, it is soft, solid, dull, sweet, heavy, cold, slimy, unctuous, and immobile.

Kapha constitutes all the solid structure of the body and is responsible for unctuousness, binding, firmness, heaviness, sexual potency, strength, forbearance, restraint, and absence of greed.

Kapha-Dominated People	Factors that Increase Kapha	Signs of Vitiated Kapha	Treatment of Vitiated Kapha
• dull in activities, diet, and speech • delayed initiation • disorderly • stable movements • well-united and strong ligaments • little hunger, thirst, and perspiration • clear eyes, face, and complexion	• salty, alkaline foods • oily, fatty, heavy-to-digest nutrients • sedentary lifestyle • lack of exercise • daydreaming • childhood • spring season • morning time • first part of the night	• drowsiness • excessive sleep • sweet taste in the mouth • excessive salivation • heaviness in the body • cold sensation • nausea • itchy feeling in the throat • whiteness in urine, eyes, and feces • deformed body organs • weariness • lassitude • inertness and depression	• pungent, bitter, astringent, sharp, hot, and rough measures • wet heat • vomiting • exercise • keeping awake • kapha-decreasing diet

From *Ayurveda: A Way of Life* by Vinod Verma

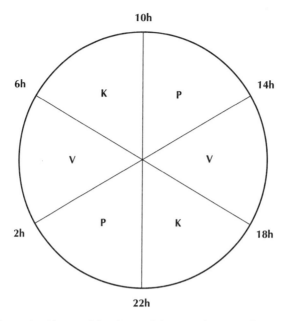

Figure 3   Hours of the day and their predominant humors.

The menstrual cycle has a strong influence on a woman's life. The different phases of a cycle during the course of a month bring alterations in her body and mind, and these changes also affect her actions and reactions. To keep good health and optimum sexual expression, she must learn to live in harmony with these changes. The two major phases of the menstrual cycle were described in the explanation of the first sutra in this chapter. The end of the secretory phase is marked by some degenerative changes and is different from its earlier part. Thus, we may divide the menstrual cycle into three main categories.

If we apply the Ayurvedic vocabulary, we will say that the postmenstrual period is slightly *vata* dominated. A woman feels free and light, and she is emotionally and physically more expressive and

Table 5   Humors in Relation to Seasons

Season	Dominating Humors
Rainy	vata
Warm and dry (summer and autumn)	pitta
Cold (winter)	kapha

Table 6   Humors in Relation to Age

Age	Dominating Humors
Childhood	kapha
Youth	pitta
Old Age	vata

Table 7   Humors in Relation to Place

Place	Dominating Humors
Forests	vata
Deserts	vata-pitta
Mountains	vata-kapha
Coastal Areas	kapha-pitta
Midlands	none

From *Ayurveda for Life: Nutrition, Sexual Energy and Healing* by Vinod Verma active. As the second week progresses, pitta begins to strengthen. At the end of fifteen days, the woman, under the influence of *pitta*, has more energy and vigor. During the third week, *pitta* slowly diminishes and *kapha* begins to increase. *Kapha* dominates during the last week or days before menstruation, and this may lead to an excess of sleep and depression. In the period immediately before and during menstruation, the three humors are disturbed to varying degrees, and a woman suffers from discomfort and minor disorders. She is relieved of all this after the menstrual release.

Let us repeat in different words the way a woman's cyclic changes are understood from the Ayurvedic point of view. Recall that *vata*, from the elements ether and air, is light, subtle, mobile, cold, rough, and all pervasive. After the endometrium layer is sloughed off, the vata-dominated period begins. A woman feels lighter not only because cells from the endometrium are shed but also because the process affects her whole body and mind.

Like any other cyclic change in nature, the process begins, expands, reaches a peak, and comes to an end. Everything begins afresh in the commencement of the new cycle. A woman feels relieved, lighter, more active, and enthusiastic. During this period, she is able to prolong the sexual act longer than at the end of the period.

During the second week, pitta also begins to enhance. The release and transport of hormones are the functions of pitta. As noted earlier, pitta is derived from fire, and among other things, it is responsible for sexual vigor. Theoretically, this period is the most fulfilling sexually for a woman. However, all depends upon the individual constitution of a person and the equilibrium of humors within her.

During the third week, the domination of pitta slowly diminishes and that of kapha increases due to the intense process of regeneration and secretion from the endometrium. As you may recall, the formation of the solid structure of the body is the function of kapha. During the last week of the cycle, kapha dominates and the endometrium gets hyperhydrated.

Kapha comes from the basic elements earth and water. The period before menstruation is marked also by a general retention of water in the body. Excess of kapha also leads to pessimistic thinking, depression, and too much sleep. A woman may feel sexually less active during this period and may have decreased sexual desire and vigor.

The period immediately before menstruation and during menstruation is generally a disturbed period. The humors are in a state of imbalance due to the degeneration of the endometrial cells and to constriction and rupturing of the arteries, followed by hemorrhage. Excess of kapha may also impair vata in certain cases by hindering its passage, and this may cause dry skin, body ache, constipation, nervousness, sleep disturbances, or some other vata-related disorders.

Blood loss during menstruation may cause weakness and fatigue and may further disturb all three humors. Due to excess of kapha, pitta may be suppressed (water and earth can extinguish fire), and women may suffer from problems related to digestion. Due to the vitiation of humors immediately before menstruation, the ojas of the body are diminished, and women may catch various infections during this period. If you carefully observe your own case, you will realize how sensitive you become and how often you have had an attack of some minor ailment during this period. Besides external attacks, chronic body ailments may also appear during this time.

We can thus see that the humors change constantly in a woman during the course of one month. Further, the individual constitution plays a role[2]—each woman's dominating humor will affect the cyclic changes, and she should pay special attention to that fact. Thus, a woman should take into consideration how her particular constitution affects her menstrual cycle. For example, if you are a vata-dominated woman, you might show some vitiation of this humor during the vata phase of the cycle. Therefore, you should carefully avoid all which enhances vata. Similarly, kapha-dominated women suffer from digestive problems and feel depressed during the premenstrual phase. Pitta domination may cause problems of digestion related to the liver and stomach during the second or third week of the cycle.

Try to avoid these problems by eating a suitable diet and taking appropriate medications. All of us—women, men, and children—should try our best to attain a humoral equilibrium by living and eating according to time, place, and our own constitutions, but women need to pay special attention during their cyclic changes.

Water retention is a problem for many women. An excess of salt, fried foods, and all other foods which make you thirsty should be avoided in the premenstrual phase or even two weeks before the cycle, depending upon the gravity of the problem. The best diet for this time should be dominant in fruits, vegetables, and juicy products. In other words, a meal with soup, salad, and fruits will be better than a piece of beef or pork with fried potatoes and cake. Also, drink plenty of water and fresh fruit juices during this period.

To maintain an equilibrium during these cyclic changes, it is essential to ensure the timely release of hormones in the right quantity. Yogic exercises to revitalize the internal organs are highly recommended. A lack of appropriate exercise may lead to related problems. The uterus is the site of release of menstrual blood, and women should take measures to rejuvenate it, particularly before conception, after childbirth, and before menopause. Rejuvenation treatment should be accompanied by revitalizing exercises.

३. काम की भावना, आकांक्षा तथा उत्तेजना में महीने के भिन्न-भिन्न भागों में दोषों की भिन्नता के कारण अन्तर होता है।

3. **Sexual desire, expression, and vigor vary during different days of a menstrual cycle, due to the change in the bodily humors.**

Let's see how the change in humors during the course of a menstrual cycle affects a woman's sexuality. Immediately before menstruation, a woman has a feeling of heaviness and may suffer from constipation or have only partial evacuation. A woman is less active, tires more easily, and generally has less sexual desire at this time. However, if appropriate measures like proper evacuation, exercise, and a liquid diet (of soups, gruels, cooked greens, etc.) are taken, sexual expression and desire can be increased during this period.

After menstruation, a woman is more active. She can have prolonged sexual activity during this period. Women who suffer from excessive bleeding or pain may feel weak immediately after menstruation and may need another week to recover until sexual desire and activity build again. Women are generally at their best during the second week of their cycle, when pitta also slowly begins to increase. This "reproductive" period is termed *Ritukala* in Ayurvedic texts. Depending upon individual cases and the age of a woman, the period may be long or short.

During the third week, when kapha begins to increase, sexual secretions are in abundance, but sexual activity may in certain cases slow down. These factors, however, are variable, especially when a woman is not healthy and has problems or irregularities with hormonal secretion.

This description of sexual capacity, vigor, and desire does not imply rigidity in sexual behavior during these periods. Flexibility and change are always possible if both partners make an effort.

४. पुरुष द्वारा यह भिन्नता अच्छी तरह समझ लेनी चाहिए तथा स्थिति को कोमलता से सम्भालना चाहिए।

4. Cyclic variations should be well understood by a woman's partner and sensitively handled.

A man who understands his woman's sexual variation can act according to the need of a given time. First, he should try to mold

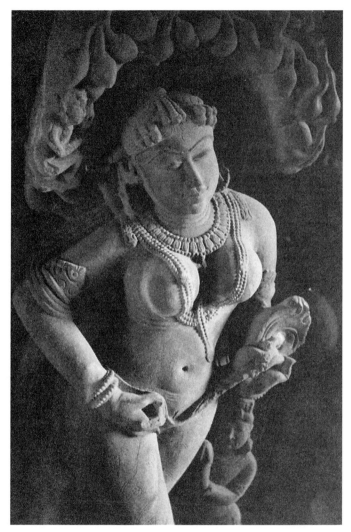

Musician.

his sexual behavior to her cyclic changes; she should help him, with patience and indulgence. Second, she should do all that is possible to keep her humors in equilibrium so that her sexual desire does not diminish completely during the premenstrual period.

A man desirous of coitus with his woman partner during her

time of lesser sexual energy should proceed with patience, indulgence, and care. The dormant sexual energy can be evoked during this period, but it requires more effort from the man and tolerance on the part of the woman. When a woman is relatively inactive during her premenstrual period, the man should approach her very slowly, with tender conversation or massage. He should try his best not to make her react, and he should do nothing abruptly and suddenly.

५. कहते हैं कि रजस्वला स्त्री को संसर्ग नहीं करना चाहिए, व्यक्तिगत रूप से विचार करते हुए इस दिशा में सावधानी से काम लेना चाहिए।

5. Some say that coitus should be avoided during menstruation; individual discretion is advised.

Many ancient texts advise avoiding coitus during menstruation. There is wisdom in this advice, since a woman's vagina is sensitive at this time, due to constant blood flow. Also, as stated earlier, a woman's immune reaction is low.

As for sexual energy, there is tremendous individual variation. Women in good health and high vitality who are expressive, outspoken, and cheerful, have a pleasant disposition, have a pitta constitution, enjoy their meals with great sensuous joy, are observant and intelligent, and are curious about knowing, learning, and exploring new things are generally the ones who have sexual desire during menstruation. However, they should be careful during coitus not to attempt difficult postures. They should not be vigorous in their movements, as the vagina and the mouth of the uterus are fragile during this period.

During coitus, the flow of menstrual blood is temporarily hindered and the vagina has its usual mucous secretion. If a woman has a strong desire and enjoys intercourse, the arteries relax again and the blood flow is restored. However, if she is somewhat unwilling and does not have a feeling of well-being, it is quite possible that the menstrual blood flow will be obstructed after the act. This has a long-term effect on a woman's health.

Women should never indulge in coitus against their own desire—especially not during menstruation. They should never force themselves to participate in a sexual act merely for the pleasure of their partners. They should not be martyrs. This sacrifice, if made frequently, may have serious consequences on their health during later years.

CARE OF THE VAGINA

The vaginal cavity can be compared to the buccal, or oral, cavity. Like this, the vaginal cavity needs constant cleaning so that it remains infection free and does not get a bad odor. It may get fungal, bacterial, or other infections if it is not regularly cleaned or if the inner natural fauna is disturbed due to the intake of antibiotics. In normal healthy condition, the vagina holds a bacterium called *Doderline*, which keeps the vaginal medium acidic by converting glycogen (a kind of sugar secreted by the vaginal cells) into lactic acid. The acidic medium is unpleasant for the growth of several pathological agents and thus helps keep the vagina infection free. However, if *Doderline* is killed due to the intake of some antibiotics or to the application of some other drug in the vaginal cavity, the natural balance is disturbed. The warm, moist vaginal environment provides an excellent terrain for the growth of many pathological bacteria, fungi, and so on. This gives rise to troubles like irritation, inflammation, and wounds.

Following are some simple methods to cure minor vaginal infections. However, if the infection persists, consult your gynecologist without delay.

1. Fresh, untreated (raw) cow's milk can help reestablish natural fauna of the vagina. It also helps to fight back minor pathological attacks. The milk, diluted with 50 percent water, should be used in a douche to wash well the vaginal cavity. This should be repeated three or four times daily until the infection is gone. If raw milk is not available, buy the least-treated form of milk from a health-food store. Yogurt with active culture is also helpful, but raw milk is more effective.

2. A cotton ball soaked in honey or ghee (clarified butter) should be placed in the vaginal cavity for several hours to cure minor irritations. Coconut oil may also be used in a similar manner.

3. Powdered licorice whipped in ghee helps cure wounds caused by parasites. Mix equal quantities of the licorice (*Glycyrrhiza glabra*) and ghee—2 teaspoons each will make enough for several days' supply—and whip these together well. With your finger, apply the mixture on the vaginal walls and around the vaginal cavity. Keep applying it several times a day and especially before going to bed, until the wounds are healed.

4. A fine paste made of crushed (or powdered) cress or mustard seeds added to an equal quantity of coconut oil can help get rid of minor vaginal infections by direct application on the vaginal walls. Make sure that you make a fine paste. Mixing 2 teaspoons of each ingredient will give you enough paste for about three to four days. Apply the paste at least twice a day until you get rid of the infection. Some people may show an allergic reaction to cress seeds.

---

६. स्त्री को चाहिए कि वह मासिक धर्म के कष्टों से छुटकारा पाने के लिए बड़े ध्यान से अपनी समस्याओं का अध्ययन कर उनके उपचार का प्रयत्न करे।

6. A woman should free herself from menstrual troubles and related disorders by studying her problems carefully and taking appropriate measures.

Many women suffer from menstrual problems. Sometimes they do not realize that their problems are related to hormones influencing their whole body. If care is not taken to maintain the equilibrium of changing humors and the balance of body and mind through appropriate exercise, diet, and other measures, a woman becomes vulnerable to all innate disorders, disorders stemming from the disharmony within the body.

Carefully study the changes in your body, and relate any of your minor troubles to cyclic changes and the context of humors. You should discuss any menstrual problems with a wise physician. You may also solve many of your minor troubles yourself by living in harmony with time, place, and your constitution. Remember always that you have to pay slightly more attention to cyclic time than men do.

Elsewhere I have already discussed how to treat most common problems related to menstruation. I want to emphasize that the fundamental causes of these troubles are improper nutrition, foods eaten at the wrong time, the lack of appropriate exercise, the ignoring of problems like constipation and indigestion, a filling of the stomach more than two-thirds during meals, a hectic mental disposition, failure to take appropriate rest during menstruation, and ignorance of the cyclic changes themselves.

Some of the preceding statements need clarification. By appropriate rest, I do not mean that you should take bed rest during menstruation. You should simply slow down your pace of life during these three to four days, get appropriate sleep, and avoid staying up late at night. A hectic way of life and a nervous disposition have a harmful effect on your menstrual cycle and may lead to hormone-related headaches. Many women suffer from migraines, which are often related to menstruation. You should learn breathing practices and yogic exercises in order to attain a peaceful disposition.

Women with jobs and with the entire responsibility for children are generally overworked and suffer from menstrual problems. They have no time to follow these suggestions. They get into a vicious circle of one trouble giving rise to another, and their sexual life suffers. Resultant familial frictions may end in divorce. A woman should be foresighted enough not to reach that exhausting state and assertive enough to share from the beginning responsibility for all household activities with her partner.

In nonpathological conditions, the extent and gravity of menstrual problems show the stress, imbalance, and emotional strain a woman has undergone during a particular month. If a woman has been working excessively or has had emotional problems or has been attending too many parties or has not been taking regular meals with appropriate nutrition, for example, the accumulative effect of all this imbalance will show up during menstruation. On the other hand, if the woman is doing yogic exercises regularly, leading a tranquil life, taking appropriate nutrition, and getting enough sleep, menstruation will also be less troublesome.

At the end of the menstrual cycle and during menstruation, the body humors are in a state of imbalance, but afterwards comes the natural equilibrium. Many believe that a woman experiences a sense of well-being after menstruation because she throws out "impure blood." In fact, the process of menstruation is a more complex cleansing process than this implies. During menstruation, the balance of the body humors is regained through such natural purification processes as the release of wind, mild diarrhea, stomach upset, and/or vomiting, strong smell in the menstrual blood or from the body, excessive sweating and urination, and so on.

The extent of fatigue and exhaustion depends upon the intensity of the cleansing process—and the degree of this latter depends upon the imbalance accumulated in the body. Women should therefore not try to cure the symptoms, which represent the reestablishing of equilibrium, but rather pay attention to the root cause of the problem.

For example, if you are a person who suffers from mild diarrhea or a strong smell in the menstrual blood or from the body, you have an imbalance of pitta. Release of wind is due to the imbalance of vata, and stomach upset and vomiting are due to a kapha imbalance. You may have one or more of these symptoms. By curing the symptoms, you will interfere in the cleansing process of nature. Rather, these symptoms should help you to diagnose yourself.

Do everything to keep an equilibrium at physical and mental levels during the menstrual cycle by paying special attention to your dominating or vitiated humor, and you will see the intensity of the menstrual troubles will decrease. Here are some general tips that should help with some of the problems just mentioned.

- Do not let your stomach become more than two-thirds full during mealtimes.

    This refers to the volume of the food, not just calories. You can overfill your stomach on simple rice and water. When the stomach is too full, there is no place for the three humors, which help digestion and assimilation. An overfilled stomach pushes out the humors and causes their imbalance, thus leading to many disorders in the body. In the case of a woman who may already suffer from minor digestive problems due to cyclic changes, overeating will aggravate the problem. Therefore, pay full attention to what you eat, how much you eat, and when you eat.

- Avoid constipation at all costs, especially during the premenstrual period.

    Make sure that you have a daily evacuation. The stool should not be hard and dry. Drinking 1 pint (1/2 liter) of hot water after getting up in the morning should cure the problem. Do not lie down after drinking it. This will ensure proper evacuation and will keep vata in order. An enema during menstruation or the premenstrual period is highly recommended for those who have painful menstruation due to constipation. However, do not make it a regular practice because too many enemas cause weakness. Try to cure constipation by altering your nutrition and drinking hot water. Constipation may also be due to some specific stress. Go to the root of the problem and try to find the reasons for yourself.

- Do not eat fried, fatty, and dried foods, especially not ten days before menstruation.

- **Pay attention to delayed and scanty menstruation or excessive menstruation, intermenstrual bleeding, or leukorrhoea.** Take appropriate measures to maintain optimum conditions (see box).

Women should avoid pain-relieving chemical drugs to get rid of menstrual pains as they provide only symptomatic relief and do not deal with the real problem. Besides, none of these drugs are without side effects.

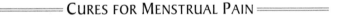

Cures for Menstrual Pain

A Note about Ingredients

Nuts should be bought raw without being subjected to any treatment and almonds always with the skin on. Be careful when you buy other herbs and spices that they are not too old. Do not buy them in powdered form. They lose their value with time and much more quickly once ground or powdered. You can easily grind them yourself with a small coffee grinder kept exclusively for this purpose, unless a hand grinder is specified. Before grinding, make sure that the herbs and spices are clean (remove any stones, etc.). Put them briefly in the sun or in a low-heated oven before grinding. For more details on the pharmaceutical properties of many of these ingredients, methods of making fine powders, decoctions, or other details concerning general preparations, you may consult my book Ayurveda: A Way of Life.

To gain immediate relief from menstrual pain without resorting to chemical drugs, apply pain-relieving oils or balms and drink a special tea made as follows: Bring to a boil and simmer for about 5 minutes 1 cup (200 ml) of water, along with 3 crushed cardamoms, 7 fresh basil leaves (or ½ a teaspoon of dried leaves), 1 teaspoonful of crushed ginger, and 3 peppercorns. Take it as is or add some black tea and steep or boil briefly. Add milk if desired, but be sure to sweeten with some sugar, since this brings an equilibrium to the spicy taste of ginger and pepper.

Almond therapy is one cure for menstrual pains that comes out of folk traditions and is used as part of regular health care in India. Eat eight to ten almonds every morning after soaking them in water during the night and then removing their skins the next day (just hold each almond between two fingers and squeeze; the skin should come off easily). It's important to start off with raw almonds with skins and to soak them in water for their medicinal value. Take them before breakfast and chew them well.

Another common cure for menstrual pains is to take half a teaspoon (5–7 gm) of kalonji (*Nigella sativa*) seeds twice daily during menstruation. In case of excessive pain, take this amount three to four days before menstruation. Crush the seeds into a powder and wash them down with a glass of warm water. Kalonji is an Indian spice readily available in Indian food shops outside India. The seeds are tiny and black, roundish on one side and conical on the other. They resemble onion seeds—do not get confused.

Half a teaspoon of garden cress (*Lepidium sativum*) seeds crushed and taken daily with a glass of warm water for three to four days before menstruation and during menstruation helps release menstrual tension and pain and also cures related digestive disorders. Cress is pitta promoting; therefore, people with this dominating humor should take care to accompany this treatment with a pitta-reducing diet. Rice, ghee, cold milk, and banana are suggested.

Dill seeds or oil (see warning below) will work much like cress. If using dill seeds, simply substitute them for cress in the preceding instructions. If using dill essential oil, take one to three drops and dilute first in water or apply to a sugar cube before eating. Whenever using essential oils, be very cautious—they are potent.

Nutmeg is also used to cure menstrual pains and delayed menstruation. A daily dose is 1/2 gram of powdered nut (about one-fourth of a medium-sized nut) or one to two drops of essential oil. (See warning above about essential oils.) Take the powder or oil as just described in the instructions for dill.

Homeopathic remedies (in each instance, a "dose" consists of 3–4 pills or pellets):

1. Chamomile is helpful if you have an early and profuse menstruation, dark blood, and pain in the lower back and abdomen. Dose: Chamomile 6X, three times a day.

2. Coffea is helpful in case of excessive excitement, nervousness, cold body, or pressure in the abdomen. Dose: Coffea 30X, twice a day.

3. Pulsatilla can help in cases of abdominal spasms accompanied by a discharge of dark clots or pale blood. The pain may change from place to place, and the stronger it is, the stronger the chills. Along with these symptoms come feelings of sadness and spells of crying. Dose: Pulsatilla 6X, three times a day.

   Nux vomica may be taken when the abdominal pain is accompanied by a constant desire to pass stool and a general feeling of dissatisfaction.

4. Platina is helpful if there is leukorrhea before and/or after menstruation, with profuse bleeding (for more on leukorrhea, see the box under Sutra 7). Dose: Platina 6X, three times a day.

5. Sulphur is a remedy when you have a headache before menstruation and colic or piercing abdominal pain later during menstruation. Dose: Sulphur 30X, twice a day.

Please note that the "X" accompanying a numeral following the name of the medicine indicates the strength of the dilution of the substance;

when you buy the homeopathic remedy, the pharmacist needs to have this indication of strength. It has nothing to do with the frequency of intake.

---

७. आर्तव में कोई भी परिवर्तन हो तो उसकी ओर शीघ्र ध्यान दें एवं बुद्धिमान वैद्य की सलाह से उसका उपचार करें।

7. Attend immediately to any alteration in the menstrual pattern and seek the advice of a wise physician.

Any vaginal infection, excessive or longer period of bleeding, excess of mucous secretion or intermenstrual bleeding, persisting pain in the lower back, and so on should not be ignored. Appropriate treatment should be undertaken under consultation of a wise physician. *Wise physician* in this sutra refers to a physician who does not treat your body like a machine. She or he examines your food habits, mental state, familial and working conditions, and other social factors directly or indirectly related to your ailment. A physician should be polite, kind, concerned, and generous with her or his time. If and when a physician diagnoses serious trouble or suggests surgery, a woman should consult at least two more physicians before making any final decisions.

If minor problems are ignored, they become major over time and may cause irreversible degeneration. So it is always important to take timely action. Women all over the world suffer from one major common factor—they are so busy taking care of the family and managing everything smoothly that they ignore themselves. Do not place yourself last in the list of priorities. Do not forget that you are the nucleus of the family. Do not derail your family by ignoring yourself; by staying healthy, you continue to provide it direction. I do not mean you should be overindulgent with yourself, but do take some time exclusively for yourself and your well-being.

══ Remedies for Irregularities ══
in the Menstrual Pattern

Delayed and Scanty Menstruation

• To encourage timeliness, take 1/4 teaspoon of crushed dill or cress seeds daily for a week before the expected date of menstruation.

• Alternatively, take a teaspoonful of sesame seeds daily, and start about ten days before your expected onset.

• Or, two to three days before the expected date, drink a decoction made from 3 tablespoons of rose petals and 1 teaspoon of anise seeds boiled in 1 1/2 cups (300 ml) water until reduced by half.

• Take 1/4 teaspoon of saffron dissolved in hot, sweetened milk (adjust amount of milk and sweetness according to taste) every day for about a month or until the problem is cured. If you do not drink milk, dissolve the saffron by whipping it into about 2 teaspoons of very hot ghee and take this after it has cooled slightly.

The problem of delayed and scanty menstruation can also be solved by enhancing the use of pitta-promoting substances in the diet. Some examples of such substances are garlic, greater cardamom (*Amomum subulatum*, not to be confused with the common, cardamom, which is smaller in size), cinnamon, nutmeg, cumin, and potatoes.

Homeopathic remedies (in each instance, a "dose" consists of 3–4 pills or pellets):

1. *Aconite* is especially useful if the delay is due to a dry, cold climate. Dose: *Aconite* 6X, four times a day.

2. *Dulcamara* is helpful if the delay is due to wet and cold. Dose: *Dulcamara* 30X, three times a day.

3. *Euphrasia* is recommended when the blood flow is very scanty. Dose: *Euphrasia* 6X, three times a day.

4. *Kali carbonicum* regulates menstruation whether it is early or late, too profuse or too scanty. Dose: *Kali carbonicum* 30X, three times a day.

Excessive Menstruation

• Take 1/2 teaspoon of crushed radish seeds with a glass of water every day for one month.

• A slightly unripe banana cut into fresh plain yogurt is another simple home remedy. Take this daily for a month or until cured. Do not add sugar, honey, or anything else to this preparation.

Homeopathic remedies (in each instance, a "dose" consists of 3–4 pills or pellets):

1. *Natrum muriaticum*, like Kali carbonicum, helps to regulate both excessive and scanty menstruation, and works well in higher doses. Dose: *Natrum muriaticum* 200X, once every other day.

2. *Crocus sativa*, made from saffron, should be taken when menstrual flow is black and slimy. Dose: *Crocus sativa* 6X, three times a day.

3. Chamomile can be taken when the blood is clotted and dark. Dose: Chamomile 30X, once a day.

4. Platina is effective when pain and a chilly sensation come with the excessive flow. Dose: Platina 6X, three times a day.

5. *Nux vomica* cures an early menstruation that lasts long and is always irregular. Dose: *Nux vomica* 30X, three times a day.

Leukorrhea

Leukorrhea is a term used to describe an abnormal, untimely, viscous discharge from the vagina and the uterine cavity. Ayurveda considers leukorrhea the result of vitiated humors, and describes four different kinds, all of which can be cured by bringing back the vitiated humor into normal rhythm.

When the discharge is foamy, pinkish, and without any smell, it is due to the vitiation of vata. Pitta leukorrhea is bluish red with traces of blood in it, and that of kapha is white or yellowish and thick. When all three humors are vitiated, the discharge is viscous (like honey) and has a bad smell.

Make a careful effort to analyze the discharge and try some of the simple remedies described below, but if the ailment persists, be sure to immediately consult your gynecologist, as it could be due to some other pathological condition of the female genital tract.

• One traditional home therapy involves mung beans baked in hot sand and ground into a flour. This flour is fried in ghee (butter fat) while constantly being stirred. At that point just enough sugar is added to sweeten the beans slightly, and the mixture is stirred until it is homogeneous. This preparation can be preserved for about two months. Take 4 tablespoons daily.

• To cure white leukorrhea, take 1 1/2 teaspoons of white cumin mixed with a little rock sugar daily.

• Make a decoction from the bark of pomegranate root, or if this is not available, take the outer part of the fruit skin. Use this solution as a vaginal douche, and afterwards, keep a cotton swab soaked in the solution in the vagina. This remedy is especially beneficial for white leukorrhea.

• Another simple remedy is to eat a slightly unripe banana with three teaspoons of ghee. This helps with vata and pitta leukorrhea.

• Leukorrhea with traces of blood (pitta) can be cured with the buds of Chinese hibiscus. Take about 10 buds and pound them in a mortar and add some milk to form a fine paste. Eat every day until symptoms disappear.

Homeopathic remedies (in each instance, a "dose" consists of 3–4 pills or pellets):

1. *Argentum nitricum* is taken when the discharge is bloody and profuse (pitta leukorrhea). Dose: *Argentum nitricum* 6X, three times a day.

2. *Arsenicum album* helps when leukorrhea is accompanied by a burning sensation. Dose: *Arsenicum album* 6X, three times a day.

3. *Iodum* is taken in case of arid discharge (irritating and pungent). Dose: *Iodum* 3X, three times a day.

4. *Ferrum iodatum* cures leukorrhea with a starchy, thick secretion (kapha). Dose: *Ferrum iodatum* third titration, four times a day.

5. *Aurum muriaticum* natronatum cures leukorrhea accompanied by vaginal contractions. Dose: *Aurum muriaticum* natronatum second titration, four times a day.

6. *Mercurius* is beneficial to cure leukorrhea that comes with a greenish secretion. Dose: *Mercurius* 12X, three times a day.

Please note that the "X" accompanying a numeral following the name of the medicine indicates the strength of the dilution of the substance; when you buy the homeopathic remedy, the pharmacist needs to have this indication of strength. It has nothing to do with the frequency of intake.

८. स्वस्थ स्त्री के रज:स्राव का रंग लाल तथा वह दुर्गन्ध-रहित होता है और दाग नहीं छोड़ता।

8. The menstrual blood of a healthy woman should be red and should not stain or stink.

There are methods of diagnosing the state of your health from your menstrual blood. Normally, the color of the blood should be red, not blackish. If you are healthy, this blood will not give a lasting stain on cloth. Healthy menstrual blood should not stink. Blackish blood indicates an excess of vata. Staining blood shows an excess of kapha, and bad odor reveals an excess of pitta. Whatever the case may be, appropriate measures should be taken to appease the imbalanced humors.

६. गर्भ निरोध का उत्तरदायित्व स्त्री और पुरूष दोनों पर है और अगर स्त्री सन्तान नहीं चाहती तो वह गर्भनिरोध के उपाय के बिना संसर्ग न करे।

9. Contraception is the responsibility of both men and women, and a woman should avoid sexual congress without the use of appropriate contraceptive measures if she does not want children.

During the reproductive period of the cycle, coitus may well lead to pregnancy. I will not go into the details of various methods of contraception here, since this is a vast subject. My objective here is to emphasize that it is the joint responsibility of men and women to use appropriate measures in order not to have an undesired pregnancy.

Since the embryo is formed inside a woman, many people think that the prevention of pregnancy is her exclusive responsibility. A woman should be assertive in this matter and should make sure that her male partner is equally involved in avoiding unwanted pregnancy. A woman who fears pregnancy and yet has unprotected sexual intercourse will often suffer body pain, stiffness, and constipation.

A woman should not get lured into having intercourse with the foolhardy idea that "nothing will happen." She should use her willpower and strength on such occasions to refrain from intercourse. She should always remember that if she has an undesired pregnancy, she herself will be the sufferer. For a woman, having an abortion is an unpleasant experience involving loss of blood and mental suffering. The body undergoes a shock. The experience may later cause a woman to develop the fear of coitus. Women should be very strong on this subject.

१०. प्रायः ४५ और ५५ वर्ष की आयु के बीच आर्तव बन्द हो जाता है किन्तु वात दोष होने से यह इससे पहले भी समाप्त हो सकता है।

10. **Menstruation generally stops between forty-five and fifty-five years of age but may cease earlier due to imbalance of the vata.**

The cessation of menstruation denotes the end of the reproductive period, which is termed menopause. Cyclic changes no longer occur. Ovulation ceases and so does the monthly formation of the endometrial layer. There is no possibility of pregnancy, and a woman no longer requires contraceptives. Menopause *does not mean* the end of a woman's sexual life.

Menopause is a gradual process related to the cessation of the formation of eggs and depletion in the release of female hormones. The premenopausal period, during which hormones are released at a reduced level, may last for several years. This reduction leads to psychological and physiological changes in a woman's body which vary from person to person, the degree depending upon the general health conditions and lifestyle of a person.

It is not possible to define these changes precisely, as any given woman may suffer from a variety of effects over a period of several years. Let us talk about some of the most common complaints and their possible remedies.

Depletion of hormones may be noticed from changes in the usual pattern of physiological effects produced by the menstrual cycle. Blood flow decreases, and the length of the cycle becomes variable. The breasts may no longer expand during the third week, as they did before. Stiffness in the body and inflammation and pain in the joints are other common features of menopause.

In some cases, the symptoms center in only certain parts of the body: a large percentage of women in my research complained of pain in the knees or lower back or cervical region. In some cases, the menopausal period may be accompanied by arteriosclerosis (calcification in the arteries) in the cervical region. Many women have pain in the upper part of the neck and the lower part of the head; others may have hot flushes or feel a sudden, momentary heat in their body even in cold weather. Such sensations may occur very frequently or only rarely. Some women feel they have suddenly begun to look old, due to dry, rough skin they may acquire at this stage of their lives due to imbalance of the vata.

Nervousness and depression are two other prominent symptoms during the premenopausal period. Some women become excessively nervous and begin to do everything in a hectic manner. They may begin to speak too much, develop anxiety for others, and begin to worry excessively. They may suffer from sleep disorders. Some women who usually have a very happy disposition and cheerful nature may lose their enthusiasm and find that all human efforts have become meaningless. Some may develop a negative attitude to life in general.

During the menopausal period, women may feel that they do not know themselves any more and cannot find a rationale for their behavior or their aches and pains. As they suffer, those around them also become victims of their strange behavior.

Premenopausal symptoms generally begin in the late forties, leading to a complete cessation of menstrual blood flow around fifty years of age. However, women who lead a very hectic and stressful life, overwork, worry excessively, and suffer from vata irregularity may end their reproductive period rather early. Vata is dry in nature. If there is an excessive disturbance of this humor, it dries up the sexual secretions, as well as the menstrual flow.

This problem must be viewed in a comprehensive way, and a woman must take a variety of steps to save herself from suffering.

The extent and the intensity of menopausal problems reflect the way a woman has been treating herself during her reproductive period. A woman who leads a healthy life by maintaining her physical and mental equilibrium is satisfied, sexually fulfilled, does not have a grumbling and complaining attitude, and may have a smooth glide into menopause.

On the other hand, a woman who has had a hard and stressful life, has not taken care of her physical and mental well-being, feels dissatisfied and frustrated, and gets tired easily may be in store for a difficult menopausal passage. Accumulated fatigue, mental tension, and neglect may all find expression at the end of a woman's reproductive period. It is like the fatigue we feel once we stop working. Before we stop, we do not realize the extent of our tiredness. But when we sit down to take rest, then we realize just how tired we are. Women should invest in their health from their younger days if they wish to diminish menopausal suffering. If you do yogic postures and breathing exercises regularly from your thirties on, and you take other measures to maintain your physical and mental equilibrium, these actions certainly pay in the long run.

Different humors dominate at different phases of one's life. Childhood is dominated by kapha, youth by pitta, and old age is marked by the domination of vata (see table 6). Menopause is the time when the dominance of pitta begins to diminish and a woman begins to enter a period dominated by vata. During menopausal changes, *all* the humors may be imbalanced, and the body's energy levels may go down. If appropriate care is not taken, various innate disorders may arise.

Many of the health problems of menopause are vata problems. Nervousness, sleep disorders, rough skin, arthritic pains, a hectic lifestyle, and excessive worrying are all symptoms of vata imbalance (see table 2). Hot flushes are due to vata-pitta vitiation. Vata is mobile and works as a distribution and communication system of the body. Its irregularity may also cause the accumulation of pitta. Besides, during the premenopausal period, the release of hormones is highly variable. Release of hormones is the function of pitta-kapha. Due to variations in their release, these humors may vitiate, causing depression and excessive heat in the body, especially in the head region.

Menopausal problems may start as early as the late thirties in some women, but a large majority show symptoms around their mid-forties. Alterations in menstrual pattern, hot flushes, a feeling of the worthlessness and meaninglessness of life, and depression are all typical. Some women find themselves extremely unreasonable and illogical, and unable to do anything about these states. Others have fits of anger that make them wonder at their own behavior. Some feel they have lost all control over themselves, while others get extremely nervous and insecure, and suddenly begin to dress fancily and apply cosmetics heavily.

Some women may begin to complain of the sensitivity to cold, various aches and pains (specially in the back), stomach upset, and a general feeling of restlessness. Others suffer from insomnia, hypertension, palpitation, extreme weakness, and low blood pressure. Some begin to put on weight, without any change in their food habits. Besides these, other nonspecific symptoms may arise which cannot easily be designated as ailments.

In former times, some cultures developed ceremonies that included therapeutic measures meant to handle menopausal problems. These ceremonies often included the intake of drugs of natural origin, as well as certain other regimens. Through these ceremonies, women decreased the sufferings of other women.

In our modern, technological age, where unrelenting activity is a way of life, and we eat generally vata-promoting food and do many other things to disturb the vata, menopausal problems have grown more intense. Besides, modern medicine has been the domain of men, who seem unable to understand the problems women have to face. Modern medicine does practically nothing for the management of menopause.

It is of primary importance that you become aware of menopausal problems, accept them as a genuine health hazard, and do all you can to cure them. It is essential to prepare yourself in advance to face this difficult period of your life. Many women suffer very intensely during these years, and this period may mark the onset of an ailment for them. This mostly happens to those who ignore their health and other problems during their thirties because they are professionally engrossed or extremely involved in bringing up their children, or both.

For example, some women may ignore a deteriorating relationship with their partner or their minor health problems or the changing relationship with their children. They may also accumulate problems concerning an imbalance between their profession and family life. They keep on tolerating these hazards for years. Suddenly, during the premenopausal period, their tolerance diminishes and they become very impatient. Those around them are generally incapable of comprehending this sudden change, which leads to further misunderstandings and an unpleasant atmosphere.

Try to think of all these possible consequences far in advance; do not go on postponing problems when you are still in your thirties. Attain the ability to anticipate the future and always face the fact that you will need both mental and physical energy for the difficult years in your forties. Accumulation of subdued difficulties of life may otherwise make a mountain within you which may well erupt like a volcano during those sensitive years.

When the premenopausal period arrives, follow minutely any symptoms or changes occurring in you at physical and mental levels. Do not ignore them or discard them. As for emotional changes, be understanding to yourself and try to make others around you comprehend your special situation by assuring them of its temporary nature, due to the "change of life" as it is sometimes called.

Generally this facet of life is rarely discussed in the family, and most children and their father interpret the woman's changed behavior as a sign of aging or mild eccentricity. Proper education about this theme is absolutely essential for the well-being of others in a woman's family as they also suffer in the process. In an extended family system, women help women and these problems are efficiently handled. However, in nuclear families, there is a need for this education so that the various facets of a woman's life are well understood and others can help her go through this perturbed period.

A regular practice of yoga strengthens body and mind and provides wisdom. Purification and revitalization of the uterus should be done regularly in your forties (see box in Part IV, Sutra 2). It is also the time when you should take rejuvenating products to keep your humors in equilibrium and the *ojas* (vitality and immune response) high. Pay special attention to your diet, and get rid of irregular eating habits. Eat a variety of fresh vegetables and fruits, and take plenty of liquid food like soups, gruels, and fresh juices. Use your mental strength, yogic breathing, and concentration practices to maintain your equilibrium.

Mental strength is something which is developed with constant practice over a period of time. It is a tremendous asset which helps us lead a fulfilled and enriched life. Keeping control over one's mental activities and directing the mental and spiritual energy to the desired direction is learnt with constant training. It is not different than learning other things in life. It is difficult to develop mental strength during the times of crisis. Therefore, in the present context, I suggest that you should prepare yourself in advance for facing menopausal problems so you can go through this phase of your life smoothly.

Ayurvedic methods for rejuvenating the uterus should be followed from time to time, especially after childbirth. The ethnic Indian tradition knows of many preparations recommended for the symptoms of premenopausal periods. These preventive methods have saved women from many major ailments in their later years. Perhaps we can take advantage of this ancient wisdom and follow some of their prescriptions.

PRESCRIPTIONS FOR THE
ONSET OF MENOPAUSE

Besides the general rejuvenating products described on the following pages, women should also take some other food supplements at the onset of menopausal symptoms. During winter, take 1/4 teaspoon of crushed cress seeds every other day.[3] During summer, take a glass of asparagus Sharvat (syrup mixed with water) daily. The method for preparing this is described in the box in Part III, Sutra 2. Eat eight to ten almonds every day before breakfast. They should be soaked and peeled, as described earlier in the box under Sutra 6.

If you get frequent hot flushes, avoid pitta-promoting foods and take a decoction of some bitter herbal teas every day for a few days (such teas include wormwood, gentian root, bitter gourd [karela], and neem). You should take some purgatives from time to time for maintaining an equilibrium of pitta. (Almost anywhere in the world, there are herbal mixtures available for this purpose.) Needless to say, coffee, an excess of black tea, tobacco, and alcohol will enhance heat in the body. The problem of hot flushes can also be solved by taking the rejuvenating products with carrots, apples, and so on (described in Part X). If this problem is ignored and it worsens, it may result in hypertension, palpitation, vertigo, and so on. If you suffer from these, do not begin to take strong chemical drugs immediately to cure these, as doing this might further complicate the fundamental problem, which is basically a temporary imbalance. It has often been observed that many women may not suffer so much from the menopausal problems as from the inappropriate treatment of the symptoms arising from them. For example, some begin to take drugs to cure hypertension or insomnia and get symptomatic relief from these problems. In the process, they toxify their bodies or get addicted to some of these drugs. They get into a vicious circle and finally remain on drugs all their lives.

Ashok tree bark is very beneficial for women in many respects. An Ayurvedic alcoholic preparation made from its bark is called Ashokarishata. This is a very effective cure for problems occurring during menopause. However, it is difficult to get a good preparation of this. Some *vaidyas* (Ayurvedic physicians) make their own medicines on a small scale, and these are often not commercialized.

Homeopathy has proven to be very useful in alleviating menopausal problems. Carefully note your symptoms, make a list of them, and see a homeopathic physician. Do not hesitate to mention all your symptoms, even those you may feel are subjective. When the onset of pain, stiffness in joints, a general feeling of being unwell, depression, and so on occurs between the ages of forty and fifty, it most probably announces the onset of menopause. Symptoms should be immediately attended to and an appropriate cure taken. These minor troubles in the beginning may cause prolonged suffering if they are not attended to in time.

If the symptoms are primarily depression related, homeopathic treatment provides the best cure. Consult a homeopathic physician and discuss the details of your particular case. Following are some well-known remedies, according to the symptoms:

Please note that the "X" accompanying a numeral following the name of the medicine indicates the strength of the dilution of the substance; when you buy the homeopathic remedy, the pharmacist needs to have this indication of strength. In each instance, the "dose" consists of 3–4 pills or pellets.

1. *Amyl nitrosum* is taken when there are flushes of heat with anxiety and palpitation. Dose: *Amyl nitrosum* 3X, four times a day. (*Amyl nitrosum* 3X is available only with a prescription in the United States.)

2. *Ignatia* is beneficial for women who are showing hysterical tendencies, irritability, and depression. Dose: *Ignatia* 30X, twice a day.

3. *Aconite* is useful in subjects with anxiety and other related symptoms like lack of sleep, fearfulness, and indigestion. Dose: *Aconite* 6X, every four hours.

4. *Sanguinaria* should be taken when a woman has burning in the palm and soles, congestion, cough, and heartburn. Dose: *Sanguinaria* 6X, twice a day.

5. A combination of pulsatilla and lachesis is given to cure multiple problems occurring during the menopausal period. This remedy is very effective and cures depression, dryness in and around the vagina, weakness, withdrawn behavior, and so on. Dose: Pulsatilla 30X, three times a day for four days. After a gap of four days, a similar dose of Lachesis 30X is taken for four days. Then repeat Pulsatilla for four days, and so forth, until symptoms improve.

---

११. आर्तव बन्द होने से स्त्री की काम भावना में अन्तर नहीं होता किन्तु आर्तव समाप्ति के पहले का काल स्वास्थ्य के लिए प्रतिकूल होता है तथा इसके लिए उपचार और चिकित्सा की आवश्यकता होती है।

11. The cessation of menstruation does not affect the sexuality of a woman, though the premenopausal period is generally hard and may need appropriate treatment and care.

Many women are terribly discouraged at the onset of menopause and associate it with old age and an end to their sexual life. Do not take it that way. Menopause marks the end of one of your exclusive and major privileges—the creation of a being—but not your sexuality.

Nevertheless, menopausal problems handled improperly *can* bring an end to the sexual life. For example, unattended depression and various pains hinder the desire for sex. Some women begin to take tranquilizers to cure their depression and sleep problems, and finally become addicted to them. Most of these medications have an adverse effect on the desire for sex and sexual vigor.

You must remember that the body, like the mind, also does not forget. Taking better care of yourself and living in balance and harmony with your environment is making an investment in good health and long life. Menopause is one period in which the neglect during your younger years may well display itself.

PREPARATION FOR MENOPAUSE

It is advisable to prepare yourself well in advance for menopause so that it does not give rise to disorders, and your sexual expression and energy remain unhindered. I suggest that women should begin to follow the instructions given below around the age of forty.

1. Do regular yogic exercises, especially those recommended for rejuvenating the uterus.

2. Try to take vata-decreasing measures such as massage, enemas, warm baths, and appropriate nutrition, which help keep this humor in equilibrium.

3. Also keep your pitta and kapha in control. Do not eat excessively pungent or sour foods. Avoid using too much coffee, tea, or tobacco. Eat more fresh vegetables and fruits than cooked and fried foods. Try to reduce the intake of meat and replace it with more dairy products.

4. Pay attention to your weight. Some women may put on weight during the premenopausal period due to disturbed humors and water retention. If you do put on weight, do not go on a radical diet, as your body needs nutrition to deal with all the physiological changes taking place. Maintain a limited and appropriate diet, and try to lose weight with yogic exercises.

5. Begin a regular practice of breathing and concentration exercises. This will teach you to control your mind. The latter will help you get out of your depression and negative feelings. The concentration practices will also help you to get rid of nervousness and sleep disorders (see Parts VI, VII, and VIII).

6. During the menopausal period, there may also be a disharmony at the level of subtle energy due to several major changes taking place in the body. I suggest you make an effort to harmonize the subtle energy with the concentration exercise given below. (Before starting this exercise, read and absorb Parts VI, VII, and VIII of this book.)

First you need to know the body movements and breathing exercises outlined in Part VI. Then attempt some of the concentration practices outlined in Parts VII and VIII, coupled with the breathing and body movements. Once you have mastered this, begin to concentrate on each of the principal energy points in the body—the chakras (see Part VIII, Sutra 9 for details). After the purification of the principal channels with *pranayama*, the yogic exercises for vital breathing (see Part VI, Sutra 10), begin to concentrate on the muladhara chakra, repeating its mantra on the night of full moon. (The muladhara chakra is the first of the seven energy centers in the body. Located at the anus, this chakra has the mantra Lam, and it represents the element earth. It governs the sense of smell.)

Concentrate on the elemental form of the chakra, earth, and on the sense of smell associated with this energy point. Slowly, try to concentrate only on the sound of the mantra, forgetting its significance. Do this practice a few minutes in the morning and a few minutes in the evening every day until the next full moon. On the night of this full moon, proceed on to the next chakra. Every time, before beginning, you should repeat the mantras from the previous chakras a couple of times before you come to the mantra of your month. Do this practice until you have reached the sixth chakra. After the sixth chakra, begin once again from the first. Make this practice a part of your life during the menopausal years.

7. Take uterus-rejuvenating products during the premenopausal period; take aphrodisiacs according to individual need (see Part X).

नारी कामसूत्र के तीसरे भाग की इति होती है। इसमें
आर्तव और काम के सम्बन्ध के विषय पर
प्रकाश डाला गया है।

**This brings to an end Part III of *The Kamasutra for Women*,
describing the relationship between menstruation and
sexuality.**

PART IV
*P*regnancy, *C*hildbirth, and *S*exuality

. . .

चौथा भाग

गर्भ और प्रसव का काम से सम्बन्ध

. . .

Oh, the lucky one, may the milk flow from your breasts like the
four oceans and be beneficial for the growth of your little one!
Oh, the fortunate one, like the gods attain longevity after drinking
nectar, may your baby also live long by drinking your nectar like milk!
—*Sushruta Samhita*

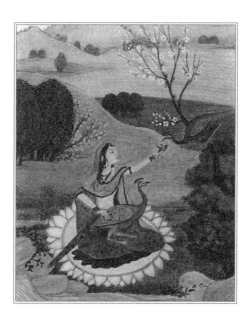

९. गर्भावस्था तथा प्रसव, यह दोनों स्त्री जीवन की महत्त्वपूर्ण घटनाएँ हैं तथा इनका काम से सीधा सम्बन्ध मानना चाहिए।

1. Pregnancy and childbirth are important events in a woman's life, directly related to sexuality.

The periods before, during, and after childbirth form a critical time, and women should be careful that events during this time do not adversely affect her sexuality. She needs full cooperation from her male partner. Pregnancy is the result of their togetherness, and all its consequences should be shared by both of them. Since the woman has to go through the physical part of creation, the man should provide her with psychological support, comfort, and assurance. Let us see step by step, the specificity of different periods related to pregnancy.

Before pregnancy: The period prior to pregnancy requires both physical and mental preparation. A couple who wants to have a child should thoroughly discuss their postchildbirth life, including the responsibilities and work the child will bring into the relationship, along with beauty and happiness. Generally, couples avoid talking about these matters, with the result that the woman has to carry most of the burden. Overwork may make her remote from herself, and her sexual expression diminishes, sometimes becoming a cause in the break-up of the family structure.

Women in whom the quality of motherhood is very dominating—who are emotional and anxious to have children—do not pay heed to more practical aspects and the related responsibilities. This category of women should be particularly careful and proceed with equilibrium and wisdom. A woman should not think about only the joy of having a baby but also about her responsibility towards her partner and his participation in bringing up the baby.

Before deciding to get pregnant, a woman must ensure that she has a healthy body and an infection-free uterus and vagina. With the help of some yogic exercises, she should revitalize her uterus before conception and take the required products for its rejuvenation.

Pregnancy: During pregnancy, a woman should be especially careful, since her habits, behavior, way of life, and thinking will directly affect the child. She should do all to ensure her baby is born physically healthy and mentally strong. Pregnancy is a state of physical oneness with her baby, and therefore she can influence him or her in many positive ways. A peaceful, healthy baby will make her life easier. A nervous baby who wakes up at night and suffers from many ailments will take a large part of her energy, leaving her physically exhausted. In such cases her sexual expression will be hindered, and her sexual vigor and enthusiasm will be considerably reduced.

Childbirth: Nine months of pregnancy prepare a woman well enough for the arrival of the baby and of motherhood. She learns to live with the developing being inside her. She eagerly waits for this major event of childbirth. Some women become anxious and impatient, while others are fearful. A woman should try to keep her mental equilibrium and make every effort to get rid of any anxiety or fear. She should regularly do breathing and concentration practices (see Parts VI and VIII) to gain mental strength and to prepare herself well for the upcoming event.

After childbirth: This is a complicated and difficult period for a woman. She is weak and fragile during this time, and she has responsibility for a baby who is initially totally dependent upon her. In addition, her male partner has expectations about renewing their restricted sexual life. She may feel that this is all too much for her. She may do what she absolutely has to (caring for and nursing the baby) and ignore or develop an aversion towards her sexuality if she is unable to manage this overwhelming postchildbirth period.

२. गर्भधारण करने से पहले स्त्री को चाहिए कि वह स्वस्थ जीवन बिताये, योगाभ्यास तथा औषधि द्वारा अपने गर्भाशय को निर्दोष, जोड़ों को लचीला और मन को सुदृढ़ बनाये।

2. During the prepregnancy period, it is essential to lead a healthy life, to do yogic exercises, and to take rejuvenating products to make the uterus healthy, the joints loose, and the mind strong.

A woman should achieve good health even before she conceives. Leading a healthy life here means keeping your humors in equilibrium by living according to your constitution, time, and place. Disturbances of humors should be cured by taking appropriate measures. I strongly suggest that a woman apply five different types of inner cleansing methods for the purification of her body. These methods are described in Part VI. She should eat a balanced diet containing a large variety of ingredients that is not dominated excessively by any one particular taste. For example, it should not be extremely sweet, salty, sour, sharp, or astringent.[1] If you are healthy before you conceive, your *ojas* (vitality and immunity) is high, and the hormonal changes that bring a temporary state of imbalance in the body immediately after conception will affect you less and reduce your suffering.

Besides purifying the body with inner cleansing practices, take measures for rejuvenating the uterus before you decide to get pregnant. Some simple recipes for this purpose are described in the box below and in Part VI, several yogic methods are described for developing strength of body and mind. A woman should follow these practices regularly for at least three months before becoming pregnant. Revitalizing your uterus with the yogic exercises prescribed for this purpose creates a good home for your baby, who has to spend the first nine months of her or his existence there. The yogic postures will also invigorate a woman in general and help loosen her joints, paving the way for a smooth delivery.

It is also necessary to develop mental strength and power of concentration before conception, for several reasons: to influence the formation of the baby and her or his behavior, to ease the childbirth itself, and to help generate a smooth flow of milk and a peaceful influence over the baby afterwards.

PURIFICATION AND REJUVENATION OF THE UTERUS

Here are some of the Ayurvedic recipes for purification of the uterus:

1. Cress seeds (*Lepidium sativum*) are available in most parts of the world, as cress salad (garden cress) is a common food. In India, it is also cultivated for fodder for horses and camels. For purification of the uterus, take 1/2 teaspoon of the crushed seeds with 1 teaspoon each of ghee and rock candy crystals. A therapy involving this treatment every day for about twenty days is especially beneficial after childbirth, and it also promotes breast milk.

2. The stigma of the the flower of *Crocus sativus* is called saffron. A rare and expensive spice the world over, it has proven therapeutic value in curing delayed and scanty menstruation. To purify the uterus, take 1/8 teaspoon, dissolved in hot milk or whipped together with some ghee and sugar, daily for four weeks. In northwest India, this treatment is given to a woman after she has given birth. (Note: Sometimes curcuma is sold as saffron in the West, so be sure you get the real thing, which is nearly 200 times more expensive than curcuma. It is not sold in powdered form, but as tiny, bright orange fibers, the dried stigma of the flowers of *Crocus sativus*.)

3. A decoction made from bamboo leaves, taken every day for a month, can also purify the uterus, although such leaves can be found only in some parts of the world. To make such a decoction, take water equal to four times the quantity of bamboo leaves you have, and boil the mixture on low heat half-covered or with a porous lid until reduced to one-fourth of its original volume. Strain the decoction, preferably through a thin muslin cloth, before using.

4. In northeast India, various products from the Ashok tree are used for contraception as well as fertility. The classical Ayurvedic medicine made from this tree is called Ashokarishata.

5. Asparagus purifies the uterus and is also an aphrodisiac. If you make a sugar syrup from its decoction during the growing season, you can preserve it for a year. To 4.5 pounds (2 kilograms) of asparagus, add 8 quarts (8 liters) of water and boil over low heat until the mixture is reduced to one-fourth its original volume. Filter the decoction and add 2 1/4 pounds (1 kilogram) sugar. Reduce by boiling until it is half the original volume. When this syrup gets cold, add 1 ounce (30 grams) of freshly crushed cardamom and 1/3 ounce (10 grams) of pepper. Two tablespoons of this mixture are recommended every day. This mixture can be made into a cold drink by adding chilled water to it. Take it for at least one month; this preparation enhances breast milk and is also an aphrodisiac.

6. Another simple method for purifying the uterus is to take 1 1/2 teaspoons of crushed cumin mixed with an equal quantity of rock candy crystals. This general tonic purifies the uterus and cures white leukorrhea. It is also an aphrodisiac and increases milk. Therefore, it should be taken especially after childbirth—daily, for thirty days.

---

३. गर्भवती होने पर स्त्री के शरीर में दो आत्माएं निवास करती हैं, उसको चाहिए कि अपने मनोबल से अपने अन्दर विकसित हो रहे जीव से अनुरूपता बनाये रखे।

3. After conception, the two souls in a woman's body mutually influence each other; she should exert her mental power to harmonize with the being inside her.

In the ancient Indian tradition of Ayurveda, it is believed that the embryo is produced from the Self, or *jiva*, which is the source of life. It is jiva which is the cause of consciousness. "Jiva entering into the uterus and combining with sperm and ovum produces itself in the form of an embryo. . . . The same foetus, by lapse of time attains the stages of childhood, youth and old age gradually. . . . The embryo, in a process of development, cannot grow without a factor other than the Self, as a sprout cannot grow from a non-seed."[2]

Soul is the cause of consciousness, while the body is the medium for consciousness. When conception takes place, the baby's soul is there, even if the body is not yet formed. That is why, in this sutra, we talk about a woman having two souls.

A baby's condition and circumstances of birth, positive or negative attributes, basic constitution, innate personality, and so on, depend upon his past karma. But an embryo is not yet capable of developing his present karma, since his medium of consciousness, his body, is not yet developed. Nevertheless, the impressions of his past deeds (*sanskara*) influence the mother. Similarly, the karma of the mother influences the baby's formation and personality. The mother is capable of controlling her present karma with her power of discretion and will. She should try her best to follow all prescriptions for having an easy childbirth and a healthy and peaceful baby.

Pregnant women usually manifest certain characteristic personality traits. Modern medicine ties these traits to hormonal changes. Most traditional societies, however, believe that these characteristics mirror the personality of her would-be child. For example, if after pregnancy she begins to feel peaceful and calm, this is traceable to the past deeds (and the basic or inborn nature) of the embryo. Or if she feels angry and aggressive, this also reflects the sanskara of her future child. Often a woman acquires other qualities during pregnancy for which she cannot find any rational explanation, including sudden changes in her emotions, likes, and dislikes. For example, some women suddenly want to learn or read about something particular or become kind and helpful to the needy. Some women become irritable, angry, or unkind, or even develop a desire to steal something or break fragile objects. Women may also develop certain kinds of strange fears, hesitations, or other emotions.

Generally, women get confused by such peculiar feelings, which they often do not share with others. I have cited only some examples here, but women experience a large diversity of emotions. Some women also feel extremely good and harmonious within themselves during pregnancy; many women have told me that their pregnancy was the most beautiful time of their lives.

The awareness that there is another soul within you which influences you during pregnancy will help you understand yourself better and help divert your thoughts and actions in a positive direction. Keep control over your emotions; keeping your mind free from the negative feelings which may dominate during this special period requires tremendous effort and constant practice. The effort is easier if you were well prepared in the period before pregnancy.

Harboring negative feelings during pregnancy may upset others around you, especially your male companion. Negative feelings always beget more negative feelings and, hence, contemptuous surroundings. An unpleasant atmosphere added to the discomfort of pregnancy will only lead to a decline in your tolerance and patience. Your irritable behavior will negatively affect your baby and may also cause problems during childbirth and hinder the flow of milk. If you have prepared yourself well before your pregnancy, you may comprehend better the reasons for your behavioral changes and be in a better position to exercise control over yourself.

From the very beginning of the pregnancy, stay aware of the other soul inside you, and always divert your feelings towards its well-being. Out of the five fundamental elements, ether and air are responsible for the formation of the foetus. A pregnant woman should concentrate on these two elements and wish for a healthy and harmonious formation of her baby. You may make your own texts or mantras for this purpose. Here is an example:

Oh powerful ether and air, you are all pervasive. You, along with fire, water, and earth, are responsible for all we feel, touch, see, hear, and smell. I concentrate on you and pray to you for a harmonious formation of my baby. Let the baby be nourished properly, have an unhindered development, and be in comfort for nine months in the darkness of my womb. After this period is finished and its development is over, may it find its way smoothly and painlessly in the world of light.

You should try to visualize the details of the individual body parts of the embryo and pray daily in the above manner for their right formation. Also train your mind and energy towards the development of positive personality traits in your baby. Whenever you feel tense or disturbed, or you feel that the being inside you is restless, go to a quiet place and practice pranayama (see Part VI, Sutra 10). Take the power of your *prana*, or vital energy, to your embryo, and concentrate your mind on the embryo. Tell it to calm down, console it, and caress it by putting your hands gently on your abdomen. Also try to involve your partner in this communication with the baby.

If you feel excessively angry, aggressive, or overwhelmed by other emotions, tell yourself that this is not good for your baby. Use your best efforts to divert your attention and calm yourself.

In brief, keep a constant watch on yourself during your pregnancy, and use your mental power to positively affect your baby.

४. गर्भावस्था में शरीर के तीनों दोषों का अनुपात बदलता रहता है,
अतः अपने तथा बच्चे के भावी स्वास्थ्य के लिए उनका सन्तुलन
बनाये रखने का अत्याधिक प्रयत्न करना चाहिए।

4. **During pregnancy, the body humors are constantly changing; for long-term health of both mother and baby,
a woman should do all she can to maintain humoral
equilibrium.**

A pregnant woman should eat a light and balanced diet. She
should eat products that promote the equilibrium of the three
humors in her body and avoid those substances that cause imbalance.[3] For example, she should eat more vegetables such as carrots,
turnips, zucchini, and salad greens, as well as mung bean soup (or
chicken soup for nonvegetarians), milk, ghee, and yogurt. However, yogurt should not be taken in excess and never in the evening
or at night. She should not eat heavy meats like beef or pork in con-
junction with fried potatoes. If she eats these meats at all, she
should have small quantities, along with rice cooked with some
ghee. She should avoid ingesting excessive amounts of spices,
and garlic and onions should be taken in moderate quantity.
The use of fresh ginger cooked with other vegetables is highly
recommended, since ginger helps bring the three humors into
equilibrium.

A preparation of mixed vegetables, rice, and a little ghee, along
with spices such as cumin, anise, ginger, and pepper, is recommended. Liquid food such as soups and gruels are also good. Eat
a variety of fruits regularly. Do not eat too much of anything, and
instead include different ingredients in small quantities in your
diet.

Do not eat excessively oily or fatty foods, and avoid fried foods.
However, do not avoid vegetable and animal fat completely. Use
ghee for cooking and vegetable oils (olive, sunflower, or corn) on
salads. Do not use rapeseed oil. Avoid repeatedly eating foods or

nutrients with one dominant taste such as sweet, sour, pungent, astringent, sharp, or salty. Excess of a particular taste makes the food unbalanced in terms of the humors. During pregnancy, regularly drink a cup to a pint of hot water after getting up in the morning, and take a walk after that, to ensure regular evacuation. Constipation or partial evacuation during pregnancy can cause many problems for both mother and foetus. Many women suffer especially from constipation during the later period of pregnancy. However, drinking water and eating a wholesome diet will save you from this problem. Besides, the practice of drinking hot water will keep the vata in equilibrium.

Imbalanced vata is very dangerous for the foetus. Dry, cold foods, preserved foods, overwork, a hectic lifestyle, staying awake at night, improper evacuation, talking too much or too loudly, emotional excitement or fear may all cause imbalance in the vata, which is responsible for the formation of the foetus. Coffee, cigarettes, alcohol, and other drugs should not be taken. Excessive use of black tea should be avoided; in its place drink very mild black tea or herbal teas. Do not take cold drinks with caffeine or other chemicals, and avoid bottled fruit juices, and all other preserved food or foods kept in the refrigerator for longer than four to five hours. Drink water or freshly pressed fruit and vegetable juices.

A pregnant woman may suddenly have a strong desire to eat something particular. It is quite possible that the desired food may not be wholesome and may cause imbalance of a humor. The Ayurvedic recommendation is to fulfill an intense desire of a pregnant woman even if the product involved is unwholesome. "When the desire is too intense, even the unwholesome thing may be given to her, added with the wholesome, with a view to satisfying her desire. By suppressing the desire, the vata gets vitiated and its movements inside the body may cause destruction and deformity in the ensuing foetus."[4]

======= CURE FOR CONSTIPATION =======

Constipation is a constant problem with pregnant women, and it causes a lot of discomfort, especially during late pregnancy. Besides keeping the habit of drinking warm water in the morning, the following are some simple recipes to cure constipation during pregnancy.

1. Take 2 ounces (50 grams) each of raisins and figs and 1 ounce (25 grams) dried rose petals. Pound them in a mortar and make a paste. Take 1 to 2 teaspoons of this mixture every night before going to bed.

2. Two medium-sized baked apples or 4 ounces (100 grams) prunes cooked in 1/2 cup (100 ml) water for ten minutes may be taken daily to ensure proper evacuation.

A pregnant woman should get appropriate rest and sleep. She should strictly avoid noisy, stuffy, and smoky places and refrain from lingering in places where people are smoking and the atmosphere is loud. Getting appropriate rest, however, does not mean that she should become lazy and do nothing. Strenuous and tiring work should be avoided; women who work outside the house should arrange for themselves quiet and peaceful evenings, with their male partners doing household duties. Some time for themselves for complete relaxation is essential. Women with strenuous professions—medicine, law, technical or scientific work—should arrange partial alteration in their duties for this temporary period at their places of work. A hectic lifestyle during pregnancy can create vata imbalance and may prove damaging for a growing baby.

I highly recommend a regular (weekly) light body massage during pregnancy. The abdomen should be massaged tenderly, with great care. A professional massage is not essential; a family member or friend should be able to give a massage meant for relaxation and the appeasing of the vata. You may also massage yourself on your hands, feet, head, and neck, and follow it with a hot shower or bath. Avoid washing with cold water, even in the summer.

Imbalance of the pitta during pregnancy can cause disorders in the foetus. Sudden hot flushes, a red complexion, and hot sweats even in winter are signs of vitiated pitta, which should be appeased with plenty of liquids, especially cold and sweet drinks. Fresh carrot juice, cold water with fresh lemon juice and candy sugar, papaya, freshly made rice and wheat preparations, and cold milk are some of the nutritional measures to cure disturbed pitta.

At a very later stage of pregnancy, nearly all women feel the symptoms of an excess of pitta. This, in fact, is a sign of the pre-delivery period. To help speed a past-due delivery, women can start a pitta-promoting diet at this stage, including potatoes, garlic, sesame seeds, dill, and fenugreek—but only under the direct supervision of a physician, licensed midwife, or other qualified person.

A pregnant woman should not sleep excessively or be lethargic. If she feels tired despite a good sleep, has a sweet taste in her mouth, and feels fatigued with little work, she may be suffering from kapha imbalance. This may cause deformation of the body parts of the embryo and may lead to a difficult and painful delivery. A pregnant woman should not submit to laziness, but always go for a walk and do some light yogic practices. The vitiated humor can be brought to rights by eating hot and spicy foods, reducing the amount of sleep, taking a hot bath or other form of wet heat, and going for walks or doing other moderate physical exercise.

Cure for Sickness during Pregnancy

It is very common for women to feel sick during the early part of a pregnancy. If appropriate care is taken before conception and a woman is very careful about her diet, this problem may not arise or it may limit itself. However, its intensity varies from person to person, and it may vary in the same person during different pregnancies. Following are some simple remedies and preventive methods to manage this problem.

1. Always keep some cardamoms with you, and if you feel slight discomfort, chew the seeds. You should also chew the seeds after your meals. Cardamom keeps the three humors in equilibrium and will bring your pitta back into balance. If you do not like the taste of the cardamom, you may chew it with some rock candy crystals.

2. Take 4 ounces (100 grams) of cumin seeds and 1/2 ounce (15 grams) of salt crystals, and drench this mixture in freshly squeezed lemon juice. Mix it well and let it dry. When you feel sick, take some of these seeds.

3. Make a syrup by dissolving a teaspoonful of rock candy crystals in a glass of water with two powdered cloves. Stir this well and drink it when you feel sick.

4. Avoid using refined sugar during this period, and use rock candy crystals to sweeten your drinks.

5. Freshly pressed fruit and vegetable juices help cure the problem. Make sure that the juice is not too sour.

6. Pomegranate has stood the test of time as an aid for this problem. Eat some ripe fresh fruit when you feel sick. Do not eat unripe fruits, as they may cause distension.

7. Homeopathic remedies

   a. Ipecac 30X should be given twice a day to cure the sickness accompanied by vomiting immediately after you get up. Dissolve two pellets in 4 tablespoons of water, and take 2 tablespoons each time.

   b. *Nux vomica* 30X should be given in a similar fashion as ipecac. It is more suitable if the person feels sick while eating or immediately after eating.

   c. *Natrum muriaticum* 30X should be given if there are symptoms like loss of appetite, stomach acidity, and excessive salivation. This should be given in water, as described above, for three days and then should be repeated at an interval of three days until the sickness ceases.

---

५. गर्भवती स्त्री को अपने स्तनों का विशेष ध्यान रखना चाहिए क्योंकि वह उसके नवजात शिशु के भोजन का एकमात्र स्त्रोत बनेंगे।

5. A pregnant woman should pay special attention to her breasts, which will become the storehouse of nourishment for the baby.

A slow development of the breasts is another important phenomenon of pregnancy. A pregnant woman should consciously follow this development and every day find a few moments to concentrate upon her breasts. Putting her hands on her breasts, she should say something like this: "Now, I am nurturing my baby with my blood, but once the baby is out of my womb, you will be responsible for feeding it and ensuring its growth. I wish for your harmonious development and a smooth flow of healthy milk after the baby is born. The way mother earth feeds all creatures in this universe, you will feed my newborn. As a river flows, so may the milk flow from you. Let it be plentiful, nourishing, and regular so that my baby can drink with ease."

Women should breast-feed their babies. A lack of breast-feeding may have ill effects on both mother and child. The ancient medical literature of India emphasized the role of breast-feeding in maintaining vitality and immunity in the child. Modern research has proved that mother's milk contains antibodies that provide the newborn with some passive immunity. And the absence of breast-feeding is also harmful for the mother. A new mother's body has prepared for this particular purpose and needs this specific outlet. Without it, a woman may feel unfulfilled or may suffer from a feeling of guilt or from blocked sexual energy. So for her long-term health and happiness, she should make every effort to ensure a proper and healthy flow of breast milk.

६. गर्भावस्था में स्त्री को अपनी कामेच्छा से अनभिज्ञ होकर अपना सारा बल एवं ध्यान अपने भावी शिशु की ओर नहीं लगाना चाहिए।

6. A woman should not ignore her sexuality during pregnancy by making her unborn baby her sole occupation.

Both man and woman cause a pregnancy. However, the woman experiences pregnancy alone. She should make it a point to include her partner in the experience at every step, but in a subtle way, not by simply discussing her unborn baby all the time. She should take a balanced view of her new situation, remembering that the baby is one part of her life but that there are other aspects to life that will go on as before. She should remember that her male partner is not experiencing motherhood as she is. If she is too preoccupied with her pregnancy and suppresses her sexual expression, her male partner may become insecure. During this delicate period both should make a special effort to increase mutual understanding and to grow together. On his part, the man should accept that her sexual activities will slowly diminish and come to a temporary halt a little before and after the birth of the baby.

During pregnancy, a woman should avoid vigorous sexual movements, as well as making love from the side or in a bent-down position. All these may result in vata imbalance, causing suffering to both mother and foetus.

Sexual activity itself during pregnancy depends upon the condition of the woman. Some women who are having problems should probably avoid intercourse during this period. Some Ayurvedic texts suggest this in a blanket way. I do not recommend such generalizations, but believe that to avoid complications, it is best to proceed with discretion and understanding.

The essence of this sutra is that a woman should keep her balance in the new situation: her child fulfills one aspect of her being, but there are other important facets to her life as well. Equilibrium is important not only for a woman's sexual life and partnership but also for her own psyche.

७. स्त्री को चाहिए कि वह अपनी मानसिक शक्ति से अपने आप को प्रसव के लिए तैयार करे जो कि एक दर्द, विच्छेद तथा खुशी का अनुभव होता है।

7. A pregnant woman should direct her inner strength towards preparing herself for childbirth, which is an experience of pain, separation, and pleasure.

Nature provides enough time to prepare a woman for motherhood. Some are very nervous about this event, and others are anxious to deliver and resume their normal appearance and activity. Try to keep your equilibrium and gather all your inner strength.

When we mention the pain of childbirth, we mean not only the physical pain during delivery but the pain of separation. The foetus has become part of the mother during the nine months of pregnancy. Once born, the baby is another human being, and the woman is no longer treated as the fragile host to be taken care of—people's attention has been diverted to the newborn.

A woman suffers physical fatigue and mental pain after delivery, gets a feeling of emptiness or void, and sometimes becomes depressed. All this may hinder the smooth flow of milk. Usually, the feeling of emptiness is mixed with the joys of motherhood—the pleasures of taking her baby in her arms and nourishing him or her with the natural flow of tenderness, love, and affection that comes from her at this stage.

During the last months of her pregnancy, a woman should mentally prepare for the upcoming events. She should visualize an independent human being with a different personality. Soon she will have no burden within, but the noise, cries, and demands of her little one. The arrival of the newborn may also hinder her sexual expression, for no other reason than the constraints of time. Visualization exercises during the last thirty to forty days before the estimated date of delivery will bring her a consciousness of the future and get her used to her baby as a separate being.

At the time of delivery, a woman requires the presence of friendly, trustworthy, affectionate, loving, anxiety-free women around her who can provide her with emotional and moral support. During recent years, in the West, it has become common to have the father present during delivery. I believe that the liberation of women does not lie in pressuring their male partners to witness this phenomenon. Here are my reasons: (1) Most men find it very difficult to witness this process, which creates in them a feeling of sexual aversion. (2) The best friend of the woman, her mother, or another wise lady in whom she has trust can often provide her with better support and healing touch than her male partner because he may feel too involved and upset at seeing her suffer. (3) Due to emotional involvement, the man may lose his presence of mind and lose his ability to help his partner, and she may feel bitter about his failure to do the right thing at the right time.

However, I do not mean to convey that a woman should forbid her male partner from accompanying her to the delivery room. Men who are themselves willing and keen to be at the scene, and who have mentally prepared themselves for the event, may be able to provide timely consolation and help to their companions.

When a woman is having labor pains, she should be constantly consoled. Her companions should tell her: "Keep courage. Soon you will have your baby, and all will be well once again." They should massage her hands and stroke her hair. For her part, the delivering woman should not strain herself until the pains appear and she feels an urge and pressure within her. Effort made too early is energy spent in vain.

A woman should get presents, consolation, attention, and care from her loved ones after delivery. People around her should not focus exclusively on the baby, and her partner should extend special care and tenderness at this time of need. This will strengthen the bond of friendship and love which is essential for the intensity of sensuous and sexual experience.

═══════ A NOTE TO SINGLE MOTHERS ═══════

Most of the concepts discussed here presume the family structure common to the majority of the world's population. However, many mothers bring up their children alone, either out of choice or due to force of circumstances. If you choose to be a single mother, you should thoroughly understand all the problems beforehand and picture yourself carrying the entire responsibility of bringing up your child by yourself. It is indeed a tough task. You should go ahead if you are confident in your physical and emotional strength and are prepared to sacrifice your personal pleasures, including sexuality.

८. बच्चे के जन्म के बाद स्त्री को अपना शारीरिक तथा मानसिक सन्तुलन बनाये रखने का प्रयत्न करना चाहिए तथा भावना पूर्वक बच्चे के साथ ही नहीं व्यस्त रहना चाहिए।

8. After childbirth, a woman should try to regain her physical and emotional equilibrium and not be overwhelmed by her new situation.

Life after childbirth can be a roller coaster between emotions of opposite qualities. On the one hand is the feeling of emptiness, and on the other, the fulfillment and blissful state of motherhood. To regain equilibrium after such a major event, a woman should not center all her emotions and activities around her baby. Other deeds, duties, and persons also have a place. To be a mother is only one part of her being. It should never become her sole occupation, as this can cause suffering in the long run.

Some women lose their sexual desire after the birth of a child. Their lives center around their child or children, and they become physically exhausted and emotionally empty. A conscious effort may be needed to break this single-minded condition. Children are very important and require time and attention from their mothers. Yet, from the very beginning children should be trained to be on their own. Women should not be clinging mothers; being so is bad for the whole family.

Loss of sexual desire after delivery may be a result of overstrain that gives rise to vata imbalance. Vata is responsible for sexual capacity, including the ability to sustain sexual activity. A person with vata imbalance may have sexual desire but be unable to give it a practical expression. Excessive vata imbalance can also dry the sexual excretions because of the dry nature of this humor.

९. स्तनों में दूध का निष्कासन रीति सहित करना चाहिए ; दूध की कमी बच्चे और माँ दोनों के लिये हानिकारक है।

9. A smooth flow of breast milk should be ceremoniously assured, and a lack of it is harmful to both the baby and the mother.

The breasts of some women develop regularly during pregnancy, but somehow, milk does not flow. This may be due to fear, the pain of delivering, or some other afflictions. In ancient times, ceremonies were performed before the baby was first given suck. In such a ceremony, the mother could both relax and become conscious of the act of feeding. Such rituals further provided a smooth transition from the period of pregnancy to the period after childbirth. These ceremonies were usually performed by wise, elderly women.

With changing times, people have forgotten the importance of such valuable old rituals and do not pay much attention to women who are young and healthy, yet are unable to breast-feed their babies. In holistic medicine, this inability is considered an ailment which may have serious consequences for both the mother and the child, including guilt feelings that may block her sexual energy.

A simple ceremony after childbirth can be organized by a woman's close friends or relatives. Several hours after the delivery, once she has taken some food and drink, has slept for a while, and feels a little better, she should be made to sit down in a reclining position and asked to concentrate on a vision of sprouting seeds and splendid flowers. She should think about the springtime, with flowers of every color on the meadows and hillsides. She should think of mother earth, the sun, water, and a fragrant springtime breeze, the springs of the mountainside, an oasis in the desert, or water flowing in a river. Slowly she should bring her thoughts to

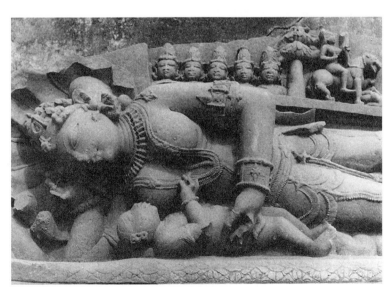

Mother and child.

her breasts, where she can visualize the flow of pure white milk from them. Her friends should show her cow's milk in a white porcelain bowl with some basil leaves or some other healing herb in it. They should tell her to concentrate on the milk, close her eyes, and visualize milk in her breasts, ready to emerge. Hold the bowl under her breasts and dip the nipples in it one by one. Moisten the rest of her breasts with milk, with the help of a cotton swab.

After this ceremony, her companions should bring the baby to her. With the baby's head on her right arm, she should give her right breast to him, with the help of her left hand. She should press her breast a little to ensure the smooth flow. Then she can repeat the same steps with the left breast.

METHODS FOR PROMOTING BREAST MILK

1. Kalonji, asparagus, and cumin are excellent for promoting breast milk. Mix kalonji, cumin seeds, and dried asparagus in equal quantities. (Dried asparagus is made from the asparagus stalk, not the root.) Powder the mixture. Take 2 teaspoons mixed with honey in the morning and evening, until you have a smooth flow of milk.

2. Twice a day, take 1/2 teaspoon of powdered dill seeds mixed with 1 teaspoon each of ghee and honey.

3. Measure 1/2 pound (200 grams) of jaggery (a kind of malt sugar); 1 ounce (25 grams) each of cumin, ajwain, and powdered dried ginger; and 3 ounces (75 grams) of peeled almonds, cut into small pieces. Heat 4 tablespoons of ghee in a pan, then add first the spices and then the jaggery. Keep stirring this constantly. Cook it for about two minutes on a low fire and then add the peeled, cut almonds. Stir it for a few seconds, and it is ready. (Heated briefly, jaggery becomes pastelike; heated longer, it becomes hard and brittle, so be careful not to overheat it.) This preparation can be preserved. It not only promotes milk but also is a general tonic that purifies the uterus and enhances sexual desire. Eat this preparation according to your digestive power.

4. Homeopathic remedies

Please note that the "X" accompanying a numeral following the name of the medicine indicates the strength of the dilution of the substance; when you buy the homeopathic remedy, the pharmacist needs to have this indication of strength. In each instance, the "dose" consists of 3–4 pills or pellets.

 a. Pulsatilla 30X should be taken three times a day to restore the flow of milk.

 b. Aconite 6X should be taken after every four hours if the lack of milk is also accompanied by fever, hot and dry skin, and frequent thirst.

 c. Coffea 30X three times a day may be given if there are symptoms like nervousness and excitement.

९०. बच्चे के जन्म के कुछ समय पश्चात स्त्री-पुरुष को अपनी पारस्परिक मैत्री तथा काम भावना को सावधानी पूर्वक नया मोड़ देना चाहिए।

10. After childbirth a couple should consciously give a new turn to their companionship and sexuality.

The sexual life of a couple during pregnancy and after childbirth can never be like it was before, and some partners are very much disheartened with this change. They lose interest in each other. The new situation should be handled with great wisdom and care, and this is only possible if both the parents participate equally in the activities of the newborn and share the perils and joys of this new experience. The woman should not be overinvolved with her baby, nor too possessive about her or him. She should not think that she is the only one who can do things in the right way for the little one. She should encourage her male partner to participate in all activities concerning the child. At the same time, she should always remind herself that there is another dimension to her life besides motherhood and another person who would like to share with her these facets.

For his part, the man should not leave the mother and the child to their fate, thinking that his duty is limited only to bringing in the money. Such a pattern is less common now anyway, as more and more women are also participating financially. Whatever the case, a man must participate in bringing up the baby from the very beginning for the sake of a full sexual life, equilibrium, and harmony. A man must remember that a woman has a natural bond with the baby, while he must build it after the birth.

Many men think their relationship with the child begins only at a later age. They also believe their relationship is limited to playing and having fun with the child. With such an attitude, they will never build a profound relationship with their child. Besides that, the company of a baby or child brings peace and tranquility into the lives of men, too often dominated by stress. Being with a very young human being may also allow their own quality of motherhood to find its expression.

A sexual partnership is not something static: it can unfold in many different dimensions. It is not detached from other parts of life, and it can be fulfilling and rich only if a couple grows together, experiencing the diverse facets of life at various levels of existence and consciousness. Sharing different levels of being such as birth, death, sickness, and success helps two people unfold in various levels of sexual experience.

If a woman has any sexual problem after childbirth, it should be immediately attended to. Vata disequilibrium should be controlled with measures such as enemas, massages, and appropriate nutrition. A man should handle this situation delicately and patiently.

Men are generally impatient to renew their sexual life and are overenthusiastic. Women need more love, care, and delicate handling at this stage. Remember that the situation is different from what it "used to be." Life acquires another style and rhythm with a baby. Some women, when they do not have an appropriate sexual response to the enthusiasm of their male partners, feel discouraged and think that childbirth has diminished a part of their sexual urge. Such a notion only makes them more nervous, and the problems can take on a serious dimension, as they start avoiding their male partners. This makes things worse.

A woman should probably wait five to six weeks after giving birth before having intercourse.

RETRACTION OF THE VAGINA

After childbirth, or with age, the vaginal opening may become enlarged. This may be subjected to treatment for bringing it to its original size. There are several recipes for this in various ancient treatises on sexuality. I have chosen a few for their ease of use, even though the first two recipes require plants largely unavailable outside of India at this time. The increasing export of Ayurvedic preparations gives me hope that this will soon no longer be the case.

1. Make a paste of lotus, along with its stem, by crushing it and adding a bit of milk. Make nutmeg-size tablets from this paste, and leave one in the vagina for an hour or two. (If fresh lotus is unavailable, you can substitute a mixture of dried root and seeds in equal quantities: to make a paste, grind the mixture to a fine powder and then add the milk.)

2. Make a paste out of the seeds of talmakhana (*Asteracantha longifolia*) by crushing them and adding water. Apply this to the vaginal walls for several days. This plant is not readily available outside of India.

3. Take the nuts from three or four tamarind seeds. (This process can be difficult without practice, because the thin brown shell surrounding the white nutmeat is very hard. The best way is to first roast the seeds for minute in a hot pan, and then let them cool before you attempt to remove the shells.) Make a fine powder from the nuts by using a coffee grinder or a stone hand grinder. Make a still finer powder by passing this through a cotton cloth (see my book *Ayurveda: A Way of Life* for details on how to make fine powders). Now create a fine paste by adding a very little water and pounding this. With your finger, apply the paste to the walls of the vagina and leave this overnight. Repeat as required. You can store this paste in the refrigerator for several days.

---

११. अपनी काम शक्ति पुनः प्राप्त करने के लिए स्त्री को बच्चे के जन्म के पश्चात् स्वास्थ्यवर्धक तथा बाजीकरण द्रव्यों का प्रयोग करना चाहिए।

11. Use revitalizing products and aphrodisiacs after childbirth in order to regain sexual vitality.

After childbirth, a woman is very prone to vata vitiation, and if she doesn't take care, she may suffer from various vata disorders. Besides, her vitality and general immunity (ojas) are low after childbirth. In addition to her fragile state, her little one demands work and attention from her. Selected nutrition and appropriate care and medication will revitalize her. There are two aspects to this revitalization. One is to bring the body's humors back into equilibrium and the vitality up to normal. The other is to revitalize the organs involved in the growth and birth of the baby. In Ayurveda we call this the cleansing process.

The new mother should rest for at least two weeks after the birth and make every effort to maintain her mental equilibrium. She may feel pain and stiffness in her body, and she may also feel restless and nervous. A warm enema with vata-decreasing drugs will help. The mother should apply warmth in other ways as well, and avoid exposure. She can use breathing exercises to regain strength and equilibrium, and two weeks after delivery, do yogic exercises to get her body, inside and outside, back into shape and to get rid of the extra weight.

A postdelivery period that is not appropriately managed can lead to several long-lasting health problems and set off a chain reaction of disagreeable events. A nervous, confused, and unwell mother transfers her negative energy to her baby, who will have bad digestion and become restless, fueling a vicious circle of panic in the mother and and the father.

A person with disturbed vata may desire sex but not have sexual vitality. If your sexual expression is hindered or obstructed, do not panic. First, bring your vata into equilibrium; then take some aphrodisiacs to enhance sexual energy (see Part X, Sutra 8). These should cure you quickly.

In summary, taking care of yourself after childbirth is just as important as taking care of your baby.

नारी कामसूत्र के चौथे भाग की इति होती है। इसमें गर्भावस्था तथा प्रसव के सम्बन्ध में प्रकाश डाला गया है तथा प्रसव के बाद के हितोपयोग के बारे में बताया गया है।

This brings to an end Part IV of *The Kamasutra for Women*, depicting the relationship between sexuality and motherhood.

PART V
The Three Dimensions of a Woman

· · ·

पाँचवा भाग

स्त्री के तीन रूप

· · ·

With their tenderness and love, may all the men in the world learn to awaken the creative and wise dimensions of women around them.

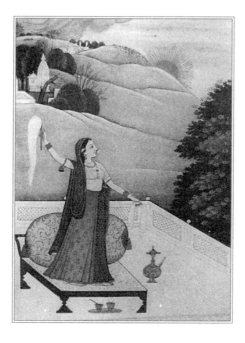

९. स्त्री के भिन्न-भिन्न रूपों की गहराई तथा शक्ति के सब पहलू समझ लिये जाने चाहिए।

1. The intensity and strength of the different dimensions of a woman's nature should be understood at all levels.

Women are fundamentally stronger and more intense than men: stronger and more intense in their emotions and experiences, in their creative as well as destructive power, and in their sensuality. This is meant not at the superficial, physical level, but at many different subtle and abstract levels. Modern psychology and psychiatry usually do not take into account these differences between men and women and in the process commit grave errors in health care. Most of the norms in these fields are developed by men, who treat all human beings from their point of view, without recognizing the subtle dimensions of a woman's personality.[1]

Still more chaos is created when women are deprived of certain fundamental rights to which all citizens of every nation should be entitled, without sexual discrimination. In certain parts of the world, women are still fighting for their basic rights to vote, to drive, to have a bank account, and to do many other trivial things. They forge ahead in this fight with the slogan of being "equal" to men, which unfortunately gives rise to a fundamental fallacy. Men and women are different in their nature and should not strive to be "equal" to each other in the various physical, mental, subtle, and spiritual dimensions of their being. To create harmony between the two sexes, and to maintain peace in our universe, we must try to understand and act upon these differences with wisdom and discretion.

२. नारी के अस्तित्व के तीन रूप हैं, निर्माण, विनाश तथा विवेक।

2. Creation, destruction, and wisdom are the three dimensions of a woman's being.

These three dimensions should be understood at the various perceptual, subtle, and spiritual levels of existence, all of which are interrelated, interconnected, and interdependent (Fig. 4). As an example, let's take the menstrual cycle. Every month, new cells are formed in the uterus, then sloughed off. Here is creation and destruction at its clearest on the apparent, perceptual level. But this physiological phenomenon also has its mental manifestation, giving rise to different sexual and personal behavior at different times of a woman's cycle. Just before menstruation, she may be tense, depressed, aggressive, unreasonable, uncertain, or nervous—all destructive aspects of a human personality.

In nature, everything is cyclic and a certain degree of destruc-

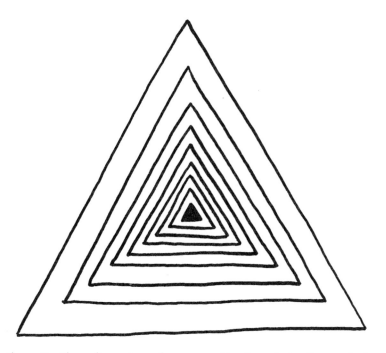

Figure 4   Three dimensions of a woman. Creation, destruction, and wisdom are represented in this drawing. Triangles within triangles show the various subtle levels of existence. The innermost triangle represents the cause of being—the soul.

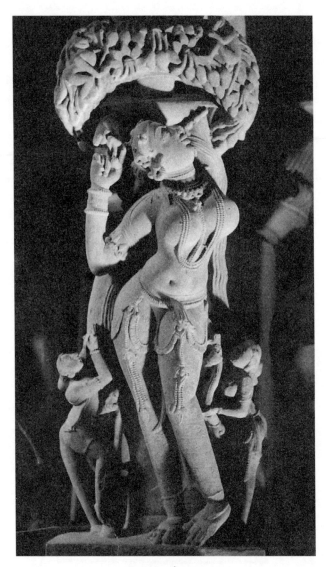

Dancing figure.

tion is essential for creation. Old leaves fall and make place for new ones. Everything is constantly changing; everything has an end sooner or later. But this end is not the end of the phenomenal world, since the new replaces the old. A basic balance is essential between these two qualities. In our times, we face environmental disasters because, with our deeds, we human beings have interfered in the natural ecological balance between creation and destruction. The destructive dimensions of a woman should be accepted and allowed a fruitful outlet. Otherwise, it will express itself as obstinacy, anger, madness, depression, aggressivity, selfishness, and so on.

Woman's ability to procreate distinguishes her from man, but this ability should not be interpreted in a limited manner. The procreative nature manifests itself in patience, sacrifice, tolerance, kindness, care, protection, and stability—qualities that are a part of her innate nature, whether or not she has offspring. Yet if a woman emphasizes only these qualities and suppresses the destructive dimension, this dimension may find another, unexpected and possibly disastrous outlet. The following folktale illustrates the importance of balance between creation and destruction at the cosmic level:

> *Once upon a time, human beings annoyed the gods, and the gods cursed them by ordering the god of death, Yama, not to carry out his duties. Soon, all creatures and human beings on the earth stopped dying. The planet became enormously crowded, dirty, and unlivable. Diseases spread as sick people did not die. Chaos reigned. Realizing the gravity of the situation, the sages went to the god of death and requested him to resume his duties— otherwise, there would be only misery and disaster on earth.*

A woman's third dimension is wisdom. To be wise means to possess a sense of discretion, a discriminating and intuitive knowledge, insight, stillness, and balance. When a woman uses her mind and her will to maintain an equilibrium and balance between her creative and destructive urges, wisdom increases.

In patriarchal societies of the world, the creative dimension of women and its attributes is accepted and sometimes venerated, while the destructive side is not accepted at all in most cultures and religions. The resulting imbalance leads to disharmony and chaos, women become dissatisfied and unhappy, and, as mothers, they create weak and vulnerable progeny. Complicated problems disturb the entire social structure.

३. तीनो गुणों के अनुपात की भिन्नता ही त्रिरूप का कारण है।

3. The three dimensions are constituted by differing ratios of the three fundamental qualities.

As discussed in Part II, the fundamental difference in the nature of man and woman is due to different ratios of male and female principles which themselves manifest different ratios of the three fundamental qualities. *Sattva* and *tamas* dominate the female principle, while *rajas* dominates in the male. Men and women both have male and female principles, but also in different proportion.

Rajas dominated by sattva gives rise to the creative dimension. Attributes such as patience, sacrifice, tolerance, kindness, care, protection, and stability are its manifestations.

Rajas with the domination of tamas gives rise to the dimension of destruction. Positive aspects of this dimension are renewal of the old, the tendency to replace, refresh, to forget bad experiences, and so on. Negative aspects are possessiveness, depression, aggressivity, irrationality, uncertainty.

Sattva, on its own—the quality of stillness, purity, beauty, truthfulness—is responsible for the third dimension, wisdom. Sattva brings discriminating and intuitive knowledge, and the dimension called wisdom has also been termed in plainer language, the "ability to sense" or "the sixth sense."

These three dimensions are in constant flux, and variations in proportion of the three provides for endless variety in human character and behavior. Dominance of one or the other depends upon the preponderance of the female–male principle and can be changed through personal effort.

Women should try to develop their discriminative power and help men with their wisdom. Men, usually dominated by rajas, tend to be overactive in worldly affairs, losing their peace of mind, stillness, and stability. Women's sattvic attributes can help them, just as men's rajasic character can be an aid to women dominated by such destructive aspects of tamas as depression, lethargy, or possessiveness.

As noted in Part II, the Cosmic Substance has three constituent

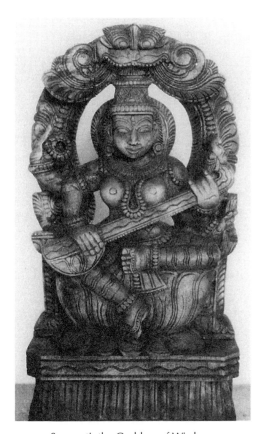

Sarasvati, the Goddess of Wisdom.

qualities: sattva, rajas, and tamas. The manifestations of these qualities are seen in the diverse forms of our existence. In relation to the body, tamas, rajas, and sattva represent the physical, the subtle, and the spiritual aspects of human existence. In the cosmic view, rajas denotes the creative principle of the universe; tamas, the devouring principle; and sattva, the principle of energy and life.

The combination of the Universal Soul and the Cosmic Substance denotes creation, which is rajas.

When these two are separated again, the phenomenal universe is dissolved, which is tamas, the devouring principle.

Sattva is the principle of purity and stillness. It denotes the presence of soul within all of us.

Just as vata, pitta, and kapha are the bodily humors, sattva, rajas, and tamas denote the qualities and activities of the mind. Thinking, planning, making decisions, and so on are the rajas activities of the mind. During sleep, mental activity is termed tamas, since the sleeping mind is preoccupied only with previously acquired knowledge and is closed to new knowledge. The sattva activities of the mind are those which lead us towards equilibrium, truth, self-restraint, control over our senses, stillness of the mind, and realization of our true self, the soul.

Sattva represents the pure element of the mind which dominates when the mind is in a state of meditation, acquires the nature of the soul, and becomes one with it. The humors and qualities affect each other. Excess of rajas may vitiate vata; excess of tamas may vitiate kapha. Sattva leads to intellect and brilliance, which are also the attributes of pitta. Vitiated vata may give rise to a hectic mental state and thus may lead to overactivity, enhancing rajas. Similarly, a vitiated kapha leads to tamas.

Figure 5 shows the interrelationship of the three humors and the three qualities of mind.[2] In normal worldly living, for sanity and good health, one needs to keep an equilibrium of these three qualities. When on the path of spirituality, one is dominated by sattva and withdraws from rajas. However, rajas is essential for our day-

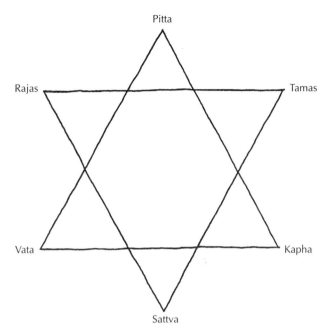

Figure 5 Interrelationship of the three humors and three qualities.

to-day living, as we must perform our duties in order to earn the means of survival. Tamas is equally important in our daily existence, as without it, we will have too much of rajas.

A yogi living in the Himalayas can afford to devote his entire time to sattva, which awakens his inner self. However, persons living in the noisy environment of a metropolis need appropriate sleep to carry out the rajas part of their lives.

The principal ailment of our modern civilization is that we have too much rajas and tamas and a lack of sattva. The dominance of greed and dissatisfaction leads to more and more rajas: people try to accumulate material goods, forgetting that everything around us is temporary, including our physical self. A lack of sattva and an excess of rajas and tamas lead to many mental ailments and sexual disorders. The rise of pornography shows that the people of our times have made sexuality into another consumers' item.

४. असन्तुलित तथा दोषपूर्ण जीवन जीने की बाध्यता अनेक शारीरिक तथा मानसिक रोगों का कारण बन जाती है।

4. Imbalance due to forced life situations may lead to physical and mental ailments.

As already stated, many societies and religions accept only the creative dimension of the woman. A woman in a patriarchal family system spends most of her time attending to the needs of family members; she gives birth to children and looks after their bringing up. All this demands patience, tolerance, and sacrifice, yet nobody pays attention to her inner needs and sentiments. She is taken for granted. Willingly or unwillingly, aware or unaware, she accepts that her life is completely centered around her family.

Meanwhile, in her body, she keeps storing tension, and in her forties or fifties this tension may take the form of a serious disease. Most vulnerable are the sexual organs, such as the uterus, vagina, and breasts. In many cases, tension is also accumulated in the stomach or lungs and may result in ulceration, cancer, or asthma.

A large number of women become victims of depression around their menopausal years, the time also when their children are becoming independent. Suddenly many women suffer from a strong feeling of being worthless.

Many times, the religious image of "a woman" stays very deep-rooted, and expressions of anger, of being assertive and free, and of allowing others to take responsibility are systematically suppressed.

Hindu tradition is quite adept at portraying the various dimensions of a woman. She is the goddess Kali, the destroyer, symbolizing time, which brings an end to all and is represented by black. She is Sarasvati, or knowledge and wisdom, represented by white. She is Laxmi, wealth and fulfillment, represented by red.

The destructive side of woman is accepted in everyday life, as is evident from these common sayings: "A wounded lioness and an angry woman are very dangerous" and "One is helpless before the stubbornness of a king, a child, and a woman."

Women should learn to accept all parts of their being. Sacrificing and doing unto others is a positive principle, but "others" also need to learn to live for themselves, as discussed in Parts I and II. Meanwhile, a woman should use her sattva quality to influence others positively; she should imbibe the qualities of stillness and peace and use her intuitive power to find her way in life, remembering that no situation is hopeless and there is always something she can do. She should not lose her mind to anger, aggression, and violence but use her energy to discover the subtle power within herself.

५. उनसे उत्पन्न उग्रता तथा विनाश दूसरों के दुःख तथा समाज में असन्तुलन का कारण बन जाते हैं।

5. Such imbalance results in destruction and violence, which give rise to misery and disturbance in society.

When a woman and the others around her accept only one dimension of her being, she may in the long run become destructive and violent (see Parts I and II). Some women adopt very dubious ways to assert themselves. Others, who crave attention, suffer from exaggerated psychosomatic ailments. Some become nagging and make life difficult for others, or adopt aggressive means to assert themselves.

For example, some women's movements declare their fight to be against men, not against the actual problems. Once when I was in the United States, I expressed to a friend of mine my shock at men's discourteous behavior. He explained that men had adopted this discourtesy as a defense against women who acted insulted and aggressive when a man held the door for them or helped them with their coat or the like.

Such aggressiveness is misguided. Trivialities such as these are no cause for a fight. On the contrary, if they are to bring about major changes, women need help and cooperation from men.

६. सत्त्व के बल से स्त्री को अपनी शक्ति बढ़ानी चाहिए तथा दृढ़ संकल्प रहना चाहिए।

6. A woman should develop her strength by emphasizing her sattvic quality and by learning to assert herself.

As noted earlier, sattva is the pure element of consciousness. Women have a preponderance of this quality, and so have a natural advantage over men. With effort, a woman can further enhance this dimension, developing her intuitive knowledge and intellect, and using this power to assert herself. In other words, she should not fight for her rights with reactionary and destructive methods, but with discrimination and wisdom.

How can a woman develop this quality of purity and stillness called sattva? Life in modern times is dominated by rajas, an excess of which gives rise to tamas qualities. People have lost their peace of mind and stillness. In former times, religions played a role in attenuating this active quality to some degree. But the advancement of technology and consumerism has weakened religion.

In the absence of religion, people should take the initiative themselves to find the means to expand the mind. Women, with their natural dominance of sattva, can play a greater role in this direction. Self-discipline, inner and outer cleansing of the body, regular pranayama (the yogic exercises of vital breathing), and concentration practice are necessary to increase sattva. Through conscious effort, a woman can rid herself of possessiveness, jealousy, attachment, greed, and so on and try to achieve a mental state of contentment.

A woman can also play a leading role in this direction by influencing her children, learning to assert herself constructively, and developing the capability to convince and influence others without losing her energy. Being assertive while emphasizing the destructive dimension only proves damaging for herself and others. Men can also develop sattva through the same means.

Why should we women be the ones to make the effort? Some women have complained about these suggestions. Their impression that they are making this effort for others is sadly mistaken. You make this effort for yourself, in order to make yourself strong and to create harmony in your life. Imbibe these qualities, and you will accumulate for yourself a priceless treasure that will help you in all walks of life.

७. परिवार तथा समाज को स्त्री के तीनों रूपों के सभी स्तरों पर मान्यता देनी चाहिए।

7. Familial and social systems should recognize a woman's three dimensions, at all levels.

Rather than creating a series of expectations built on a one-dimensional image of an "ideal woman," society must change its customs, rituals, and social norms to accept a woman in all her dimensions. The image needs to be rebuilt; in addition to the eternally kind, tolerant, and sacrificial mother, we also need to learn to face her angry, devouring self.

८. काम के स्तर पर भी स्त्री के तीनों रूपों की अभिव्यक्ति होनी महत्त्वपूर्ण है।

8. The three dimensions of woman need appropriate sexual expression.

If a given society expects a woman to express only one of her three dimensions, they expect this to be translated into sexual terms as well. In other words, she is to be giving, tolerant, and patient—a passive partner who is subjected to sex. A woman should make a conscious effort to get rid of this image and realize that it is not possible to bring equilibrium to her life unless she has balance in her sexual expression as well.

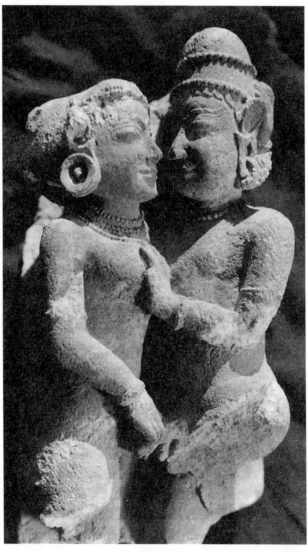

Erotic couple.

The sexual act reflects the three dimensions in the following sequence: creative, destructive, and wise. Sexual actions are creative and directed towards a definite goal. As the goal is nearly reached, a woman's destructive dimension, her devouring principle, is activated. This stage is quickly followed by a moment of pure consciousness, denoting the third dimension. The profound experience and fulfillment of the two last stages depends upon the intensity of her participation in the first part of the act (see Part XI).

SEXUAL ACTIVITY AND THE THREE QUALITIES

In sexuality, rajas is the performance of the sexual act itself, sattva is the short moment of beatitude at the end of sexual activity, and tamas comes in briefly before the experience of sattva. This latter may be prolonged through personal efforts, and the sexual energy may be channeled in diverse ways. In the absence of this effort, there is another period of tamas at the end of the sexual act, leading generally to physical rest or sleep.

६. असन्तुलन की निरन्तरता से कामेच्छा का अन्त हो जाता है क्योंकि यह तो गुणों से ही उत्पन्न होती है।

9. A continued imbalance in the three dimensions of a woman may bring her sexuality to an end, since sexuality is a byproduct of the three qualities.

If an equilibrium is not maintained for a long time among the three dimensions of a woman's being, the imbalance creates disharmony in the three fundamental qualities and in the bodily humors, and her sexual expression fades. Sexuality is governed by these humors and qualities; their imbalance leads to malfunction. At the level of the humors, sexual enthusiasm and endurance are the domain of vata, sexual vigor comes from pitta, and sexual secretions come from kapha. At the mental level we see rajas, sattva, and tamas, respectively. An imbalance at any of these three levels produces a lack of fulfillment. If this lasts, sexual interest diminishes and sexual desire slowly withers away.

१०. अपनी स्थिति को सुधारने के लिए कोई समय असमय नहीं होता, पर उसके लिए भरपूर प्रयत्न तथा अनुशासन की आवश्यकता होती है।

10. It is never too late for a new beginning, but such beginnings require tremendous effort and self-discipline.

It is possible to repair the damage caused by long-term imbalance. Never think that your case is hopeless. Instead, gather courage and make a fresh beginning, remembering that only effort and self-discipline will bring rejuvenation. The effort pays off—not only in sexual fulfillment but also for general health.

Although every situation is unique and there can be no fixed set of instructions, one thing is certain: renewal requires getting rid of excessive attachment and involvement. This does not mean you should do something such as leave your family. On the contrary, put your efforts into a constructive change. With detachment, you will learn to see things dispassionately and become able to judge your situation with wisdom. In any event, do not fall into despair. Human beings have unimaginable strength once they decide to awaken the energy dormant within themselves.

KARMA: PAST AND PRESENT

It is important to understand the relationship of karma and Ayurveda. All of us are born with and have to go through different conditions and states of health. This is due to the past karma, called *daiva* in Ayurveda. However, we can improve or worsen our conditions with our present karma, *purushkara*. Maintaining good health and relationships requires coordination between the daiva and purushkara. That means that our present karma concerning our health depends upon the conditions we already have. All of us need to pay special attention to our weak points. If I am blessed with a strong constitution and a pleasant disposition, it does not mean that I should be negligent, but rather should make every effort to maintain this state until old age. Many people think that karma implies a deterministic attitude. It is not that at all, and personal effort is extremely important. Purushkara which is the basis of all health care practices.

---

११. परिस्थिति में परिवर्तन तथा नये उत्साह के साथ कार्यों में संलग्न हो जाने से सफलता मिलती है।

11. Renewal comes easiest with a change of atmosphere and activities.

To get rid of an unhappy situation, you need to distance yourself, to look at everything dispassionately. A change of atmosphere and activities may be essential if you need to detach from the existing situation and find a new perspective.

Going away to a peaceful place for a holiday may give you time to reflect and put your energies together. Alternatively, you may learn a craft such as pottery or take up painting. These activities may give you time to better comprehend yourself and see others from a different perspective.

In troubled situations, people often talk too much with friends. Differing opinions lead to confusion and to a destructive, tamsic attitude. Talking to others is important, but ultimately it is our own wisdom and inner stillness (sattva) which should guide us. In a state of sattva, we develop the capability to see ourselves and others from a level other than that of the day-to-day routine, to appreciate the positive and beautiful within ourselves and within others.

इससे नारी कामसूत्र के पाँचवे भाग की जो कि स्त्री के तीन रूपों का वर्णन करता है की इति होती है।

This brings to an end Part V of *The Kamasutra for Women*, describing the three dimensions of a woman.

PART VI
Physical Power and Sexuality

. . .

छठा भाग
शारीरिक शक्ति का काम से सम्बन्ध

. . .

Once upon a time, the demons troubled the gods very much and these latter decided to send *Kama*, the god of love, to awaken *Shiva* from his meditation so that he could save them from the demons. *Shiva* was angered for being disturbed and he reduced *Kama* to ashes with the fire of his central eye. Henceforth, the lust became bodiless (*ananga*). Thus, lust has no structure, but it expresses itself through all the organs of the body.

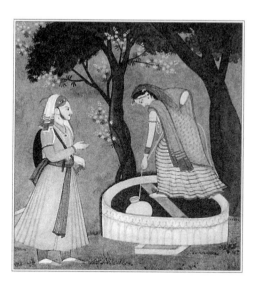

९. कामपूर्ति के लिए शरीर का हित प्राथमिक है क्योंकि यह इसका साधन है।

1. Since the medium of sexuality is the body, its well-being is a basic requisite for sexual fulfillment.

Sexuality has many dimensions, including the physical, mental, social, and spiritual. However, the physical dimension is the most basic one. The body is the seat of sexuality. The word *body* in this sutra refers to the physical self of one's being, which also includes mind but does not include the power of discretion or intellect. In other words, the body is the seat of the five senses, with the mind registering what senses perceive from the phenomenal world. We may be able to develop our intellect and achieve spiritual experience through sexuality, but the body remains the basic medium. A malaise in the body or discomfort in the mind hinders sexual expression and inhibits the intensity of the experience.

२. नियमित रूप से बाह्य और आन्तरिक शुद्धि करने से स्फूर्ति प्राप्त होती है तथा सुन्दरता बढ़ती है।

2. Both inner and outer cleansing are essential for health and beauty.

In modern times most people emphasize outer cleansing and beautification, mainly through artificial means, and few pay attention to "inner" cleansing. However, a periodic inner cleaning of the body can create a state of well-being that increases physical attraction and charm.

Ayurvedic practice recommends five types of inner cleansing methods, to be followed twice a year for purification of the body. Most important of these practices in the present context is the enema. An enema removes stiffness from the body, makes the skin smooth and shiny, and spurs activity. A woman who suffers from constipation and partial evacuation may experience abdominal tension and pain during the sexual act. If the constipation is chronic, she may also lack sexual excretions. In the case of men, an enema increases their power of retention. Enemas are not just a cure for constipation but are effective in cleaning and rinsing the intestines. They pacify vata, bring tranquility, and enhance sexual attraction. I recommend them highly for both men and women. A nonunctuous (nonfat) enema should be followed by an unctuous enema with a mixture of milk, oil, ghee, and honey.

Other inner cleansing practices of Ayurveda also contribute to general equilibrium by rejuvenating the body and enhancing vigor and strength. You must, however, follow appropriate cleansing procedures, with the right herbal mixtures and appropriate quantities of drugs. Outer cleansing practices should not be ignored either. They bring a feeling of well-being and make one attractive and agreeable.

In certain cultures, external beauty is emphasized only for women, while men are supposed to enhance their physical strength. For an intense and profound experience of sexuality, both men and women require physical attraction and strength.

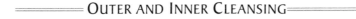

OUTER AND INNER CLEANSING

Outer Cleansing

Mouth, teeth, and tongue: While brushing your teeth, clean your tongue properly with a soft toothbrush. A dirty tongue can give rise to an unpleasant smell. Each time you eat something, rinse your mouth with water, or if that is not possible, eat a cardamom or clove to purify your mouth cavity. Chewing four or five cardamoms a day will perfume the mouth and strengthen the teeth.

Nasal passages: To clear your nasal passages for a free flow of vital air, or *prana* (see Sutra 10 in this Part), always blow your nose strongly after you shower, dip two of your fingers in mustard oil, insert them in your nostrils, and inhale. This exercise should make you sneeze and clear your nasal passages. If you suffer from a constantly blocked nose or sinuses, try the yogic exercise known as *Jalneti*.[1]

Ears: Clean the sticky secretion of the ears from time to time with a soft cotton swab. Remember to wash the outer ear while you shower; afterwards, press the upper lobe of your ears by taking them between your fingers and thumbs.

Eyes: Use mild eyedrops (preferably artifical tears or homeopathic or Ayurvedic eyedrops) for cleaning the eyes. Mild chamomile or basil teas are also recommended for eye cleansing.

Skin: Because soaps and shampoos dry the skin, give your body an occasional rub with a paste of powdered almonds and milk. Rub the paste in well, then wash it away. As for soaps, use only those prepared with natural oils and without perfume. Also, try saturating the body with oil weekly (preferably coconut or sesame or ghee), massaging it onto all parts until the skin will not absorb any more. Afterwards, a hot wet towel can be used to remove the extra oil. Be sure to shower the next day.

Head and hair: Your scalp gets very dry with the constant use of shampoos. To help counter the dryness, massage your head several hours before shampooing your hair with enough sesame or coconut oil to wet the scalp. A mild shampoo or hair-washing soap is best, and a mixture of one part lemon juice to two parts honey as a conditioner. Rinse this out.

Vaginal cleansing: From time to time, use a vaginal douche or wash your vagina using an enema bag. Best for this is a decoction of chamomile or a mixture of bitter herbal teas usually sold as liver tea in the pharmacy. Also possible is a 5 percent solution of neem oil, which can now be found outside India. For one douche, use 1/2 cup (100 ml) water per 1 teaspoon (5 ml) pure neem oil.

Inner Cleansing and Purification

Neglect of the inner parts of the body and the accumulation of dirt in them lessens one's beauty and charm and can in the long run cause ailments. What follows is only a brief description of inner purification practices; consult my book on Ayurveda for more detail, and best of all, get some practical training if possible. Do not attempt inner cleansing if you are pregnant, fatigued, or otherwise not in good health. Obese persons and those with weak digestion should avoid unction.

Fat cure and fomentation: This cure helps loosen the accumulated dirt inside you and increases the effectiveness of the other inner cleansing practices. The idea of the fat cure (or unction) is to saturate the body with an oil massage on the outside (as just described) while simultaneously ingesting fat. The quantity of fat depends upon your digestive capacity. An average recommended dose is 1 to 2 tablespoons of ghee in hot sweetened milk taken for three days at bedtime. Fomentation, the sweating process, then follows—one or even two days later—either in a Turkish bath (wet fomentation) or in a sauna (dry fomentation)—or if you live in a sunny climate, in a sunroom. After sweating, cover yourself with a blanket and avoid exposure to the air. When your body is dry, take a hot shower. (If neither a Turkish bath nor a sauna is available to you, you can take a very hot bath with one or two drops of thyme or dill oil in it and then put on a bathrobe and get into a warm bed. Thyme essential oil will burn the skin if more than three drops are added to the bath.)

The two enemas: First is the herb enema, done with a decoction of chamomile, anise, verbena, wormwood, or thyme, depending on your basic constitution. (Chamomile is good for all constitutions; while anise or verbena is good for vata-, wormwood for pitta-, and thyme for kapha-dominated ones. If none of these herbs is available, use lightly salted water.) The liquid should be warm, at the temperature you usually use for your shower. Insert it in through the anus using an enema bag while lying down on your left side with your left leg bent. Once the liquid is in, stay lying down in a relaxed position for a while, then walk around gently as long as you can hold the liquid inside. Take a rest after evacuation, and eat hot and light food, such as warm soup, sweetened rice, or cooked vegetables.

An unctuous or fatty enema should follow on the next day, with a 1 cup (240 ml) solution that contains 5/8 cup (160 ml) of milk and 1/8 cup (27 ml) each of honey, ghee, and sesame oil. Try to keep this liquid inside your body for several hours.

Purging: Take a strong herbal purgative mixture (not oils) before going to bed, causing a thorough evacuation the next day. Here are some examples of purgatives:

1. Three to four figs (*Ficus carica*) before going to bed with some hot water or hot milk.
2. About 1/4 ounce (5 grams) powdered linseed, with some hot water or milk before going to bed.
3. A tablespoon (10 ml) of castor oil.

Having liquid stool five to seven times speaks for good purgation. This treatment revitalizes the liver functions and helps cure skin problems.

Emetics: This process involves voluntary vomiting after you have consumed a prescribed liquid.*

Here is one method: Take about 1 quart (1 liter) of licorice decoction with 1 teaspoon sea salt crystals in it, or meat or vegetable soup. Incite the regurgitation by tickling in the deeper part of your throat. Stoop at about a 45-degree angle while retching; you should heave no more than eight times.

---

*Although an established part of Ayurveda for centuries, many Western physicians are uncomfortable with this, perhaps because of the prevalence of eating disorders. Please do not undertake this or any procedure in this book casually or without consulting a qualified professional.—*Ed.*

Urinary tract purification: You can purify the urinary tract by taking a strong diuretic and consuming plenty of liquid to clean out the urinary system. Diuretic herbal teas generally sold for bladder or kidney infections may be used for this purpose. Barley salts is one suggestion, or ask your pharmacist. Keep warm while taking this treatment, and eat a warm liquid diet afterwards.

Blood purification: Products such as fenugreek, garden cress, coriander, dill, basil, turmeric, and garlic are natural blood purifiers. Treatment can consist of taking 1 teaspoon of a mixture made from equal portions of each of the herbs mentioned (but omitting the garlic), in powdered form, ingested with water every day for fifteen days.

३. त्रिदोष-सन्तुलन से ओज बढ़ता है तथा इससे काम शक्ति बढ़ती है।

3. Equilibrium of humors enhances ojas, hence sexual vigor.

When the humors are in equilibrium, you stay healthy and your ojas increases. As noted earlier, ojas is the body's vitality and its capacity to defend itself from external attack. An increase in body vitality means an increase in sexual vigor. Besides, when you have more vitality, you have more sex appeal and desire, and more capacity to enjoy the intensity and depth of sexuality.

४. स्त्री और पुरुष दोनों के लिए शारीरिक शक्ति को बढ़ाना आवश्यक है।

4. Men and women should develop their physical power.

Women as well as men need to develop their physical strength for a fulfilling sexual experience. Many times, force and virility are

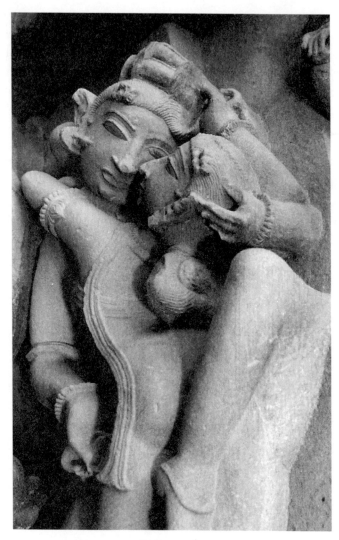

Erotic couple.

associated with men, as they are supposed to "sexually satisfy" their woman partners. Mere sexual satisfaction is a very superficial experience and does not speak for its potential intensity and depth. Satisfaction is enjoyable, it provides a momentary exhilaration, but it cannot bring you to a state involving every pore of your body, where the intensity can touch the depths of your mind and lead you to a state of pure consciousness. This state is possible only when the woman is equally active, where she is not only led but also leading. During sexual union, pleasure and joy form a chain of actions and reactions. Active and appropriate participation of one person provides an impetus to the other, and so on.

५. नियमित रुप से शरीर की मालिश करने से त्वचा की विषय भोग शक्ति बढ़ती है।

5. A regular body massage enhances one's tactile sensation.

A regular body massage makes the skin smooth and sensitive. It is a good idea to massage yourself once a week and saturate your body with oil. Use warm ghee, coconut or sesame oil, and keep applying until your skin does not absorb any more. Remove excess oil with a hot, wet hand towel, and take a bath a few hours later (or the next day). If repeated, such massages will make your skin strong, sensitive, and smooth, and enhance your sensual pleasure.

A professional massage from time to time is also a welcome experience. However, the most effective massage is the exchange of massage between partners, learned properly and done systematically.

६. सुवासित शरीर आकर्षण का कारण बनता है।

6. An agreeable body smell increases attraction.

An unpleasant or strong body odor can be a hindrance in sexual expression. Some people hide their body odor with perfumes, eau de toilette, and so on. This can suppress the odor, but it can also mix with the natural strong smell, to give rise to a peculiar odor that becomes even more of a hindrance. I advise dealing with this problem at the basic level; besides, a natural, pleasant body smell itself acts as an aphrodisiac.

It is usually pitta-dominated persons, or those with vitiation of this humor, who release strong odors from their bodies. They sweat too much and generally have an oily skin. They should pacify this humor by taking a purgative (one of the cleansing practices), and afterwards begin eating a pitta-decreasing diet with such foods as rice, cold milk, green vegetables and salads, freshly prepared wheat products, and so on. They should eat less meat, potatoes, garlic, and other strong-smelling foods. If they do eat strong foods or spices, they can chew cardamom, anise, or betel nut (the nut of areca palm).

Ointments can be medicinal and can perfume, beautify, or perform many other functions. Anoint your body occasionally with sandalwood paste or clay. These can help to cure vitiated pitta. Clay cleans the body thoroughly and sandalwood also perfumes the skin. Anointing with either of these helps to get rid of many skin toxins.

Some people do not realize they have a strong smell, since they themselves have become used to it. Sometimes, they clean themselves daily but do not change clothes. Whatever the case, do not hesitate to talk about these problems with your partner and try to find a solution. No aphrodisiac can be effective until the anaphrodisiacs are removed. For further discussion of anaphrodisiacs, see Part X of this volume.

७. इन्द्रिय शक्ति को बढ़ाने का प्रयत्न करना चाहिए।

7. Make an effort to enhance your sensual capacity.

Sexuality involves a full immersion of all five senses, so if you enhance the power of the senses with conscious effort you can intensify the sexual experience. Here, a tranquil mind and perseverance will slowly bring rewards. Increasing the capacity of the senses means awakening the dormant capacity, sharpening your sensitivity, and developing harmony with your inner self. To illustrate this idea, I want to cite some beautiful mantras from the *Rig Veda*.

May our entire group of sense organs, supporter of human life, giver of rich rewards and confidence, function perfectly in consonance with the inner self—the soul.

May our swift-moving senses, givers of happiness, bring functional perfection as the solar rays gently bring daylight.

May our entire sense organs be free from decay. May they be full of cognitional activities and devoid of malice. They are capable of receiving and remitting the rays of divine knowledge. May they be nourished to the full.[2]

You can make an effort to enhance your olfactory sensation by consciously recognizing various smells our universe offers us. Take deep breaths from a particular flower or spice, and keep the air inside you by closing both your nasal passages. Concentrate on the smell, then slowly exhale the air. Do this several times for each odor. Keep up this practice with other smells you encounter: a pine forest, wet earth, the sea, and so on.

An enhanced sense of smell helps you to establish a distinct relationship with the different body parts of your partner and will make you aware of your own body smells. You will realize that your body smells vary during different parts of the menstrual cycle and that body smells also change according to the seasons and the food you eat. Strong-smelling foods leave their odor mostly through perspiration, in the armpits, and in the case of women, in their vaginas as well.

Develop a sensitivity to various tastes in the cosmos. Do not reject new, unknown, exotic tastes without even experiencing them.

The senses of taste and smell are closely associated in both eating and sexual experience.

Try to make your voice melodious, and sharpen your auditory capacity. Listen to the natural sounds of birds, water, and wind: concentrate on them, and try to recognize them. Learn music, learn to sing, and learn different languages.

With your power to see, learn to observe the ever-changing universe of various forms and hues. Look at everything minutely and carefully. Do not just pass by trees growing along the road without observing the changes in them by season. Look carefully at the growing seedlings, and watch the buds slowly changing into blooms.

Developing the power of the senses not only intensifies sexual experience but will enrich you in all walks of life.

८. शरीर के अंगों का लचीलापन लावण्य, स्वास्थ्य तथा संभोग क्षमता को बढ़ाता है।

8. A flexible body enhances grace, health, and sexual ability.

Relaxing the body at a physical level and making it flexible depends upon your state of mind. A tense, worried, or restless mind stiffens the body immediately.

The first step for obtaining flexibility is to check several times a day to make sure that you are not in a tense or stiff sitting posture. People generally keep their shoulders, vertebral column, or abdomen tense. Regular yoga practices will be particularly helpful.[3] It is important that all your joints be flexible, including ankles, knees, hips, wrists, elbows, and shoulders.

Our vertebral column, which protects the spinal chord, is an extremely flexible part of the body. Most people spoil their beauty and physical capability by keeping the vertebrae stiff. You must learn not to limit yourself in space but to expand yourself with flexible movements like those of flowing waters or a moving snake. Such movements are good for your general health, make you look elegant, and are very beneficial for prolonging and intensifying sexual experience. They can be learned by sitting cross-legged and then bending backwards and forwards as far as you can extend yourself. Similarly, you must learn to make round movements from the base of the vertebral column. These movements can then be used during different coital postures.

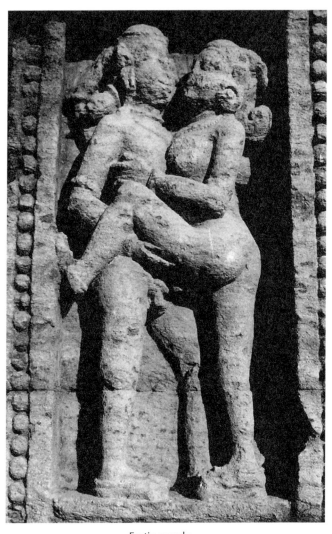

Erotic couple.

Efforts to make the body flexible and elegant not only en-hance sexual pleasure but can uncover different interrelated dimensions of our being. Sexuality is only one part of our multifarious existence, and it is interwoven with the others.

६. अभ्यास के द्वारा योगासन सिद्ध कर लेने चाहिए।

9. Develop the capacity to hold yourself in one posture with yogic practices.

Yogic postures, or *yogasanas*, help increase concentration of the mind, self-discipline, and flexibility. They revitalize the internal and external body parts. Certain postures are specifically suggested for women, for revitalizing the uterus and strengthening the vaginal muscles.

In general, the ability to sit at length in a given posture will help you make various postures during sexual union. Variations in these postures enable one to experience different levels of sensibilities in sexuality. However, this deeper sexual experience is possible only if your partner possesses an equal mastery over his body and mind. A person with a stiff body and hectic mental state may prove very disappointing in the totality of the experience. So make sure your partner gets equally trained in these practices. Generally, women are more willing than men to learn these practices. If your partner is unwilling, try to initiate him slowly by demonstrating the positive results of your new knowledge.

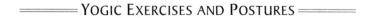

YOGIC EXERCISES AND POSTURES

General Instructions for Yogic Practices

Practice yogic postures with an empty stomach and bladder, and in the open air or with an open window, in a peaceful environment. Wear stretchable or loose clothes and use a blanket, carpet, or mat spread on the floor.

Before beginning the yogic practices, bring yourself to a calm and relaxed state. Sit down and loosen your body parts. Take a few deep breaths by inhaling smoothly and slowly and, after a brief pause, exhaling in a similar manner.

Many of these exercises and postures are not from the classical yoga. Through my researches, I have devised new exercises and positions (yogasanas) that are particularly beneficial for the exchange of sexual energy and sexual fulfillment for both partners.

Rejuvenation of Vaginal Muscles

Lie down on your back and put your arms upwards and cross them with each other (Fig. 6). Keep your legs at a distance of about 30 centimeters, or one foot. Become completely relaxed. Concentrate on your body, its form and appearance. Breathe consciously and rhythmically. Bring your attention to your vaginal cavity. Contract and relax the vaginal muscles several times. After a while, coordinate the muscular activity with your breathing. Contract while you inhale. Retain your muscles in a state of contraction while you are holding your breath. Then relax them slowly while you exhale. After repeating this several times, pause for several breaths, then repeat, but this time by widening the space between your legs as far as you can. It is more difficult to move the vaginal muscles in this posture.

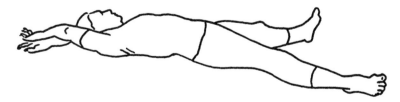

Figure 6

Benefits: As you'll see, I also recommend repeating this exercise while keeping the various sitting postures described below. This exercise strengthens and increases the sensitivity of the vaginal muscles, thus enhancing pleasure during coitus. It also prevents the vaginal opening from widening, so it's especially recommended after childbirth.

Rock Posture

Sit with folded legs so that your hips are on your heels, and slowly move your legs sideways (from the knees downward), until your bottom is resting on the floor. Put your hands on your knees (Fig. 7). Breathe slowly and smoothly. In the beginning, sit as long as you can comfortably, then slowly increase the time. Once you get used to this posture, use it as a sitting posture from

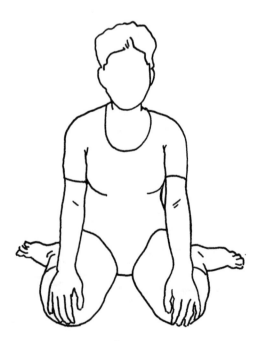

Figure 7

time to time to strengthen your body. You can also do the vaginal muscle exercises and practice *pranayama* (concentrated breathing) in this posture.

Benefits: As the name suggests, this *asana*, or posture, makes the body strong and stable and gives an erect posture to the spine and shoulders. It helps prevent hemorrhoids, strengthens the thigh muscles and ankle joints, and helps make the pelvic and knee joints flexible.

Angular Posture in Erect Position

Sit straight on the floor with your legs stretched out and your hands on your thighs. Make certain your shoulders and back are not bent. Loosen up. Slowly spread your legs as far apart as you can, and stretch out your arms to touch your feet with your hands. Bring your back as far forward as you can (Fig. 8). If your body is flexible enough, bend down to touch the floor with your forehead.

Benefits: This asana makes the pelvic joints flexible and can facilitate childbirth. It also makes the uterus flexible, making more room for the fetus. This is a good posture for the preconception period.

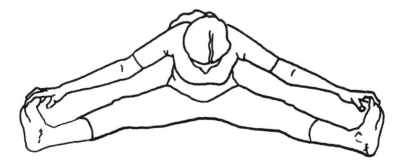

Figure 8

Angular Posture While Sitting with Bent Knees

This exercise should follow the one just described.

Straighten your back and bring your legs together by joining the soles of your feet; your knees will bend in the process. Hold your feet together with both your hands, and bring them in as close as possible by pulling them gently towards you. Your knees should stay as near to the ground as possible (Fig. 9). Once in this posture, release all the tension from your body. Sit as long as you comfortably can. Slowly increase the time in subsequent sittings.

Benefits: This posture works on the pelvic joints from a different angle than the previous two. It also revitalizes the abdominal muscles, including those in the urinogenital system. This is also a good pre-pregnancy asana.

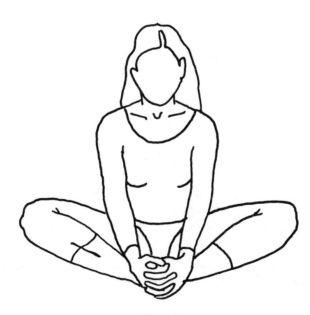

Figure 9

Angular Posture While in Whole-Body Posture

Lie down on your back with your legs together and both hands on your sides. Let your body relax, and then gently begin to raise both your legs. When your legs are at a right angle to your body, give a slight pause and bring them towards your head. Your waist will be slightly raised in the process. Place both your hands on your back to provide support as you raise your whole body upwards. Once your body is in a straight line and your whole weight is supported by your neck, shoulders, and back of your head, you are in the whole-body posture. Spread your legs as far as you can. Your breathing will be slow and short in this position.

Slowly start bringing your feet together in such a way that the soles are touching each other (Fig. 10). Bring the joined feet as

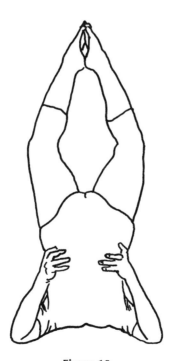

Figure 10

far down as you can, and stay in this position for a few seconds (Fig. 11). Repeat these up-and-down movements several times.

Some of you may experience the release of air from the uterine cavity while assuming this posture and making the up-and-down movements. Try to contract your vaginal muscles if you can. Your breathing will automatically follow the rhythm of your movements.

Caution: People with cervical problems or back injuries of any kind should not attempt this posture.

Benefits: This asana is beneficial for the whole body. It especially revitalizes the uterine region and makes the pelvic joints flexible, facilitating childbirth. This is another good preconception asana.

Abdominal Movements

Lie down on your back with your hands slightly away from your body. Bend your legs so that your soles touch the ground. Concentrate on your abdominal area, and move the abdominal muscles up and down. Retracting the abdomen forces your breath

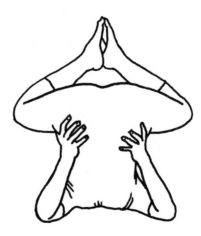

Figure 11

out. Make sure that you move only your abdominal muscles, without moving the rest of your body. Repeat five to ten times with a rest of two to three breaths between each time.

Benefits: This exercise revitalizes the urinogenital organs, regulating their functions. It also has an aphrodisiac effect.

Knee Movements

Lie down on your stomach, and spread your arms and legs a little apart. Pick up your right leg from the knee downward (the foreleg), and make circular movements with it in slow motion, in the air (Fig. 12). Synchronize one circle with one breath. Position the heel of one foot close to your hip, and begin making the circles while you inhale deeply. Coordinate your movement in such a way that you complete the circle at the same time as you finish exhaling. Now make the same movement with the other leg. Repeat the movements both clockwise and counterclockwise.

Benefits: These circles in the air strengthen the knee joints and lower back muscles, which helps you use your foot and the sole flexibly during sexual activity.

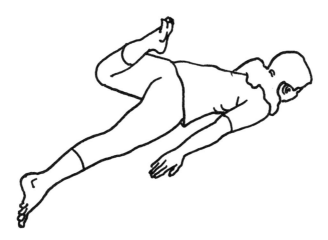

Figure 12

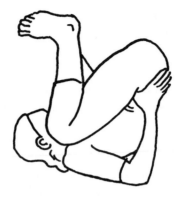

Figure 13

Folded Whole-Body Posture

Assume the whole-body posture described earlier. Bend your legs and bring down your knees in such a way that they are on either side of your face (Fig. 13). Slowly increase your capacity to stay in this posture.

Benefits: This posture is good for the whole body and makes the spine flexible. If you develop the ability to stay in this posture for a long time, you can use it during sexual union.

Frog Posture

Sit down in the rock posture, as described earlier. Bend forward, put your forearms on the ground and rest your head between them (Figs. 14 and 15). Try to contract your vaginal muscles and make up-and-down spinal movements at the same time. Take care that your posture does not alter during these movements—the force you are using should come from your back. The positions of hands, feet, and shoulders should remain unchanged.

Benefits: This posture makes all the body joints flexible. It is another useful position for sexual union.

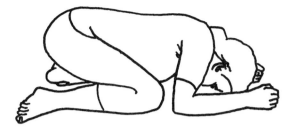

Figure 14

Pelvic-Joint Movements

1. Lie down on your back and spread your legs apart. Gently lift one of your legs as much as you can without bending your knee, and make circles in the air with it (Fig. 16), both clockwise and counterclockwise. Repeat with the other leg.

Caution: This exercise requires a tremendous amount of force, so do not do it more than three or four times.

Benefits: This pelvic-joint exercise increases flexibility, which will be useful for childbirth and for various postures during sexual activity. It helps firm the abdominal muscles, and revitalizes the whole abdomen and the large intestines. This is a good exercise before a woman conceives and after she gives birth.

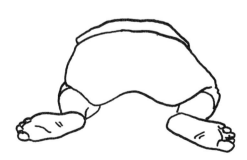

Figure 15

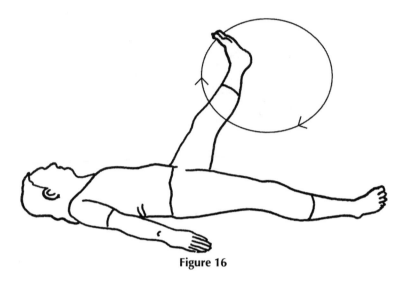

Figure 16

2. Put your leg up as just described, and then bend it from the pelvic joint in such a way that your foot is touching the ground on the other side (Fig. 17). If you have lifted your right leg, it should be bent towards the left side so that it crosses over your left leg and arm. Repeat with the other leg.

Benefits: This provides strength to the abdominal and lower- and side-back muscles. It makes the pelvic joints flexible from yet another angle, and prepares the body for yet another position during coitus.

3. This exercise is nearly the same as the one just described, and it provides the same benefits. In this one you bend your knee and touch the ground on the opposite side with the sole of your foot (Fig. 18).

4. Lie down on your back with legs slightly apart and both arms to the side. Push down your right leg without lifting it up. In this process, the left leg will slightly retract. Take care not to bend the knee of the left leg. Repeat the same with the left leg. Go on alternating the two legs, and do this in different rhythms. Dur-

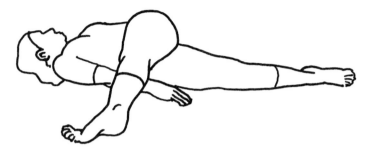

Figure 17

ing this exercise, your legs, especially the heels, will rub the ground, and the movements are made from the pelvic joints. The upper part of the body should not move.

Benefits: Besides strengthening the pelvic joints and revitalizing the vagina and uterus, these movements enhance sexual desire and can also be used during coitus.

Zigzag Posture

Stand on your knees and bend forward to touch the ground with the front part of your head. While in this position, stretch both

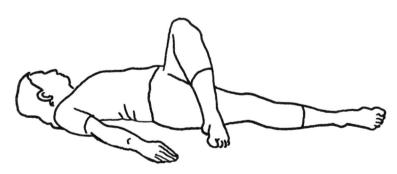

Figure 18

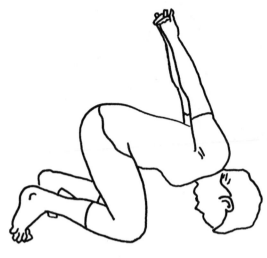

Figure 19

your arms upwards and hold both hands together (Fig. 19). In this position, your body weight is on your toes, knees, and the front part of your head. Gradually, develop the ability to stay in this posture longer.

Benefits: This asana makes all the joints flexible and enhances the body's capacity to make various sexual postures.

Sprout Posture

Lie down on your back in a relaxed position, and fold both your legs in such a way that your thighs are touching your abdomen and the knees are closer to your breasts. The parts of the legs below the knees remain upwards. Place your arms around your knees and join hands (Fig. 20)—this will press your forelegs towards your front part and will temporarily widen your vaginal cavity. In this position, the body shape looks like a growing sprout, hence the name I've given it (*ankurasana* in Sanskrit).

Benefits: This asana revitalizes the whole body and is a good one for variety in sexual postures.

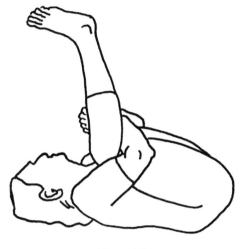

Figure 20

Flower Posture

Lie down on your back in a relaxed position with hands slightly away from your body. Lift both your legs very slowly and then spread them as far as you can without bending your knees. Hold your toes with your hands (Fig. 21).

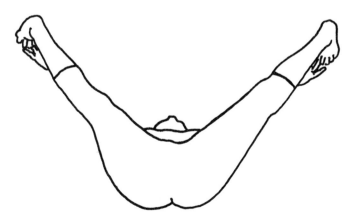

Figure 21

Benefits: This asana strengthens the abdominal muscles and makes the pectoral and pelvic joints flexible. It is another good position for sexual union.

Head-Toe Posture

I have named this position *Nakha-shikha* asana, as it involves touching the forehead with your big toe. Stand straight and loosen yourself. Lift your right foot and bring it upwards by holding it in both your hands. Bend your head a little and touch

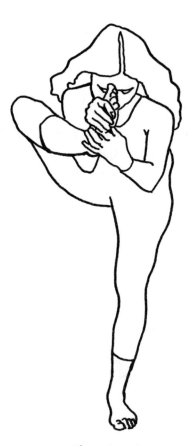

Figure 22

the big toe with the center of your forehead (Fig. 22). After a brief pause, do the same with the other foot.

Caution: This is a difficult position and requires a very flexible body. Do not force yourself. You will need training in other yogic exercises before you are able to do this.

Benefits: This position provides practice in standing on one foot while bending your body. It helps in all standing sexual positions.

Spinal Movements

1. Sit down cross-legged, put your hands on your knees, and make slow and steady circular movements with your body from the base of the vertebral column (Figs. 23–25). Your whole body from the seat upwards should move together—in other words, when you are making a backward movement, do not lend it support from your waist. The upper part of the vertebral column stays straight. Move both clockwise and counterclockwise, making the circles as big as possible.

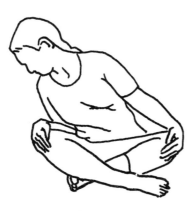

Figure 23

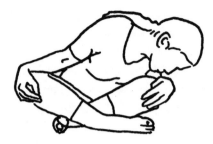

Figure 24

2. With your waist, make similar circular movements, but while standing. Put your hands on either side of your waist and move the upper part of your body in as big circles as you can, both directions, slowly and steadily (Fig. 26).

3. Sit down cross-legged, put your hands on your knees, and loosen up. Stretch your back upwards as if you were raising yourself with the help of your vertebral column and back muscles. Release this stretch slowly and relax. Make the same stretch by going up and down in a zigzag fashion, like a snake.

4. Stand straight with your feet slightly apart, and rest both hands below your waist. Look behind you by turning your waist (Fig. 27). Do not change the position of your feet or pelvis. Repeat from the other side also.

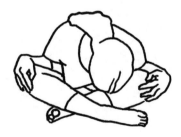

Figure 25

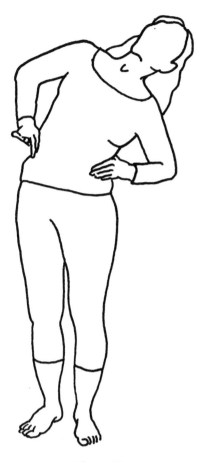

Figure 26

5. Stand straight, as just described. Make circular movements with your pelvic region. Your feet and shoulders should not move. Only the region below the waist and above the thighs should be involved in these movements.

Note: Wherever circular movements are involved in any of the exercises, you should try to make them clockwise and counter–clockwise, in circles of various sizes or in spirals.

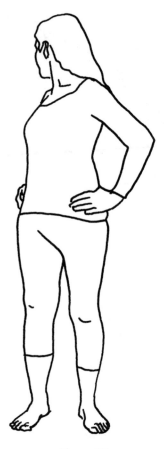

Figure 27

Benefits: All these movements make the vertebral column and spine flexible and revitalize the back muscles. They help a person make various movements during sexual union.

१०. प्राणायाम के अभ्यास से भिन्न-भिन्न स्तरों पर कामशक्ति की वृद्धि होती है।

10. Practice of pranayama increases sexual intensity.

Prana is the vital energy that pervades everything, including the air we breath in. Prana forms a link between the body and the soul. Body is the material reality of our being, while soul is the cause of consciousness. When breathing stops, the body and soul separate, bringing death. A controlled breathing process facilitates control of the activities of the mind.

Pranayama exercises include many different kinds of controlled breathing. Pranayama forms one of the eight yogic practices. It involves the progressive deceleration of the respiratory rhythm by prolonging inhalation and exhalation and by increasing the central pause of holding the breath.[4] Pranayama expands vital energy, increases general vitality of the body, and improves concentration of the mind.

A regular practice of pranayama increases stamina, sexual energy, control of impulse, and power of retention. It helps one attain a peaceful mental state and regulates the vital energy in the body. A pregnant woman should guide her vital breath for the well-being of the growing baby. Prana can also be used for healing.

During the sexual act, there are different levels of breathing from the beginning to the end. When the actions cease, the vital breath is retained deep inside, where it stays for a moment. With its exhalation comes a period of beatitude. Pranayama exercises can help prolong the moment of sexual beatitude, extend this into a spiritual experience, and provide an ability to use sexual energy for different purposes. In other words, practice of pranayama intensifies each of the steps leading to sensual fulfillment and happiness.

═══ BREATHING PRACTICES, OR PRANAYAMA ═══

For an initiation into pranayama practice, begin simply by breathing in an aware manner. Inhale very slowly and smoothly, and disperse this vital energy throughout your body. Let it flow through to the tips of your fingers and toes. After making a brief stop, exhale in a similar slow and smooth manner. After a few breaths, repeat the same by guiding the vital breath to the upper parts of your body. Feel the vital energy circulating in your head region—eyes, ears, mouth, and nose—and exhale slowly after a brief pause. In the third step, guide the vital energy to the outer surface of your body and feel it on every part of your skin. Do each of these three practices for three to four breaths to revitalize your body, your mind, and your five senses. This simple practice can be done whenever you have a brief pause from work.

Following are some exercises which you can easily learn on your own. After mastering the techniques, apply them to control the activities of your mind.

1. Sit down in a comfortable posture, preferably cross-legged. Place your hands on your knees. Loosen up, straighten your spine and close your eyes. Inhale very slowly and smoothly, and concentrate upon the prana energy you are taking inside you. When you have inhaled sufficiently, pick up your right hand and close your nostrils with your thumb and ring finger. Keep your nostrils closed as long as you can comfortably, then release them, bring down your hand to its original position, and exhale smoothly and slowly. In the beginning, the air may gush out with great force. But with constant practice, you will acquire control over it. When all the air is out, close your nostrils with your left hand, and hold the lungs without air as long as you can comfortably. Release your fingers and slowly inhale again. In the beginning you may find this difficult; but with regular practice the time for each step increases, and you will be able to do all the steps spontaneously.

2. Pranayama is useful for the purification of the two principal channels running on either side of the spine. In this case, you use only one nostril at a time, keeping the other closed.

After acquiring the pranayama posture just described, close your left nostril with your left thumb, and inhale slowly and smoothly with the right nostril. Then close the right nostril also with your ring finger, and after a while exhale by lifting this finger. Close this nostril again, and hold the lungs without air for a moment. This process cleans the sun channel, located on the right side. Repeat this eight to ten times. Do the same with the left nostril, to clean the moon channel.

3. This step involves circulating the prana energy in both sun and moon channels, and it should be attempted after purification of the individual channels as just described.

Inhale from the right nostril by closing the left with the left hand. Close the right nostril too after inhalation. After a while, lift your thumb from the left nostril and exhale slowly and smoothly. Close this nostril after all the air is out. Now, inhale from the left nostril. Repeat eight to ten times.

4. This step of pranayama involves rapid breathing. Sit in a relaxed posture as previously described, and begin to breathe very rapidly, as if you had just been running a long distance. Continue as long as you can do so comfortably. This exercise will give you a cool feeling in the head and open blocked energy channels in this region.

The three principal energy channels of the body have diverse significance at various levels. The sun and moon channels signify male and female energy respectively. At another level, they signify action and inertness, or rajas and tamas. The central channel in between these two represents sattva: equilibrium, beauty, truth, etc. The third exercise of the pranayama described above is for reaching equilibrium of both the sun and the moon channels in relation to sattvic energy. Since the sun and moon channels also represent our existence at the very fundamental level of material reality, it is essential before doing the third exercise or any of the advanced pranayama practices to purify the sun and moon channels as described in the second exercise.

After having mastered the pranayama techniques described, you should learn to develop the ability to direct prana to a desired part of the body. You will have to practice regularly, twice a day, after getting up and before going to bed. Every week, choose a part of your body to which you wish to direct your prana energy. Concentrate on that particular part of the body before beginning the practice. Then slowly inhale as if you were taking the vital breath to that part. While the vital breath is inside you, as your nostrils are closed, let it circulate through that part, then exhale slowly. You will feel some heat in the part where you are directing the energy.

Success in this practice is possible only if you have mastered the principal technique of pranayama. Your concentration should not be diverted towards thinking which finger you have to lift from which nostril.

---

१९. विभिन्न स्तरों पर अनुरूपता महत्त्वपूर्ण है और इसमें शारीरिक साम्यता सर्वप्रथम है।

11. Compatibility is important at all levels, the physical being the most basic.

Compatibility exists at many levels and involves all different aspects of a partner's existence. Physical compatibility, the cause of attraction, is at the root of sexual experience. You may be fascinated by somebody's intellect or wisdom, but if this person does not appeal to you physically, you will naturally want to refrain from any bodily contact with him. It is not the physical beauty or ugliness of a person I am referring to. These are usually limited to norms within a given society, and there are many, many other attractive or repulsive physical qualities, like body smell, cleanliness, ways of talking and eating, and so on.

People's external mannerisms reveal a lot about different dimensions of their physical being. Therefore, observe minutely before you make a choice. Good observation helps you avoid many complications and may save you from being disillusioned. If a man eats very fast, looks at his watch often, or displays other distracting mannerisms, he probably needs to learn a lot in the sexual domain. If you nevertheless find him attractive, do not expect too much at the sexual level as you begin the relationship.

Similarly, someone who is slow, takes too much time to respond to any situation, or pauses often while speaking may also not be very promising in terms of a sexual relationship. The one who talks too much and wants to impress you with his conversation, and does not even see that you are getting tired or bored, is basically insecure, and you may have a very complicated and unsuccessful sexual relationship with him.

Look also for physical compatibility with a man's dominating humor. A slightly fat person with clear eyes is kapha-dominated. This person will have abundant sexual excretions, but may not have that frequent a desire for sexual union. These types are generally home and family lovers and are committed to companionship. A vata-dominated man with slightly hectic mannerisms and rapid movements will generally be very good in admiring you and expressing his great desire for sex, but he may not be as good in performance as in talk. A pitta-dominated person generally has hot skin, may sweat a lot, and may have a strong smell. He will have more sexual vigor and energy than the previous two types.

नारी कामसूत्र के छठे भाग की यहां इति होती है। इसमें शारीरिक शक्ति का काम से सम्बन्ध बताया गया है।

This brings to an end Part VI of *The Kamasutra for Women*, on the relationship between physical power and sexuality.

PART VII
Mental Power and Sexuality

. . .

सातवां भाग
मानसिक शक्ति का काम से सम्बन्ध

. . .

He devours the world,
he is called *Kama*.
He gives with one hand and takes with the other,
he is full of intelligence and strength.
He is ever moving and is difficult to suppress.
He is a form of fire
and we offer him oblations.
—*Atharva Veda*

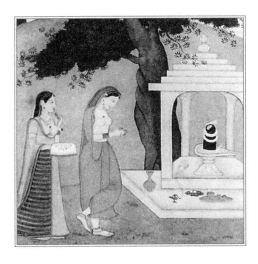

९. काम की गहन अनुभूति के लिए मानसिक शक्ति को बढ़ाना चाहिए।

1. For a profound experience of sexuality, increase your power of mind.

In some ancient Indian texts, the mind is considered to be the sixth sense. The mind registers the knowledge which the senses constantly perceive in the phenomenal world. But let us see first what is really meant by the power of the mind.

The real power of being and the cause of consciousness is the soul. The soul is without any substance. It is only energy, a part of the cosmic energy. The mind is a medium to reach this immense source of energy. The mind is, on the one hand, the cause of our involvement with the material world and, on the other hand, the path to the dormant energy within ourselves. To put this idea in simple words, we can say that mind has two forms—one which gives shape to the perception of the senses, and the other when the mind comes to a state of stillness and is no longer involved with the senses. In this latter state, the mind becomes one with the soul and is the source of power, or *shakti*.

Even during sleep, the mind has a chain of thoughts. Through constant effort and perseverance, one can intercept this chain of thoughts and bring the mind to stillness. Developing this capability of withdrawing the mind from sensuous experience and bringing it to a state of stillness is the key to mental power. A first and simple step in this direction can be taken by developing the ability to concentrate on an object or symbol. The pranayama practices facilitate the process of achieving concentration of the mind (see Part VI).

By utilizing our mental power, we can direct our inner energy towards a complete sensuous expression that results in a state of beatitude and stillness. By attaining mastery over the mind, we can direct it to prolong the experience of beatitude in sexuality.

२. मैथुन के समय मानसिक शक्ति दूसरे के मन तथा शरीर के भाव को समझने में लगानी चाहिए।

2. During the sexual act, apply your mental power to understand the physical and mental expression of the other.

Any type of communication requires concentration of the mind. During the sexual act, communication takes place at various levels, as different parts of the body interact and all the senses are involved. Only by concentrating the mind completely on the gestures, movements, expressions, and feelings of the other, can one effectively communicate and enhance the quality and pleasure of sexuality. The ability to concentrate should be slowly developed, and you should not think that you can do it during the sexual act if you cannot otherwise exercise such control over the mind. In fact, it is always important to concentrate on what we are doing to be completely with an activity at a given moment of time. Doing so increases our efficiency and capability in all domains of life, including sexuality. Effective communication during sexual activities sets in motion a chain of actions and reactions. If you are not concentrating, you cannot respond to the other's needs and be further invigorated by his or her pleasure.

३. अवरुद्ध मन:स्थिति से काम भावना का भी अवरोध होता है।

3. Mental blockage hinders sexual expression.

Blocked mental energy also affects sexual expression, even with the desire for sex. While sexual desire may compel one to begin sexual activity, a mental blockage means there is no drive to continue it. The mental blockage may be caused by any strong emotional reactions—shock, grief, anger, hatred, aversion, disappointment, dislike, and so on. A suppressed sexual desire for someone who is not accessible can also cause such blockage. If the problem is not attended to, it can give rise to serious ailments.

Diverse methods can be applied to relieve mental blockage. At the emotional level, forced crying usually helps. Shouting, singing loudly, or finding another form of strong self-expression, such as acting or painting, can also prove effective.

४. स्त्री-पुरुष को एक दूसरे के लिए एकत्व की भावना होनी चाहिए।

4. It is essential to develop a feeling of oneness with each other.

The feeling of oneness is not something you get through rational thinking. This sutra does not mean that you should continually remind yourself during sexual union that you and your partner are submerged into each other. The feeling of oneness is an experience which comes after you've attained perfection in sexual communication, which itself comes only by extensive personal efforts and by developing the ability to concentrate the mind on a single object (singlepointedness). The oneness of the male and female energy (the Purusha and the Prakriti) is the primordial cause of our phenomenal world. The experience of oneness during sexual union symbolizes the cause of the phenomenal world.

५. चित्त की एकाग्रता से तेज तथा आकर्षण बढ़ता है।

5. Singlepointedness of mind gives rise to radiance and enhances attraction.

As already said, singlepointedness of mind is the ability to keep up a state of concentration for some duration. The strength of the mind increases through repeated practice of singlepointedness, through yogic methods. This strength helps us attain sexual perfection and also lends us an extraordinary radiance and beauty.

Beauty cannot be defined merely in terms of the physical attributes of a person. We all know some people are attractive despite the fact that under defined social norms they cannot be considered beautiful. It is an inner radiance that lends them charm and beauty. The physical attributes we are born with are due perhaps to our previous karma, but each of us is capable of developing our inner energy to acquire radiance from our eternal, immutable source, the soul.

६. मनोबल के उपयोग से कामशक्ति को कल्पना द्वारा व्यर्थ नहीं होने देना चाहिए।

6. Sexual energy should not be wasted on fantasies; always control the mind.

A lack of self-control makes people dwell on thoughts about sex, wasting their sexual energy without ever having a chance to express it at an appropriate occasion. Concentrate, and fulfill your sensuality when you are indulging in sexual practice. Do not live in the time "not yet come" and waste your energy in preparing yourself in advance (in your imagination) for an event that has yet to happen. Rather, spend time and energy developing the concentration and self-control that will help you attain sexual fulfillment.

It is very agreeable to think about pleasant sexual experiences of the past or to fantasize about would-be joys of the future, but both activities diminish the power of the mind. The simplest formula to develop your power of the mind is to stay completely in the activity you are involved in. If, while you are sitting at your place of work, your mind is projected on the great event of the evening, when you are going to meet the man of your dreams, you will not only become inefficient at work but also diminish your sexual capability and expression. If you feel overpowered by such thoughts, consciously stop yourself, do some pranayama, and bring back your concentration to the work you are involved with. Some activities may seem so purely mechanical that you need not concentrate on them. If so, use this time beneficially by concentrating on a single object or your chosen symbol or mantra, and develop your mental strength that way.

The process of achieving a thought-free mind should not be limited to a session of only a few minutes. You should always try to check your wandering mind. Pay all your attention to the task you are involved with or the person you are talking to or anything else you are doing. In addition, take a deep breath and concentrate on the *ajna* chakra (see Part VIII) for a moment before starting a new task. By constantly following the activities of the mind, you will begin to learn to control them too.

There is a category of people who believe in being "sexy." Many women dress scantily, speak in a husky voice, exude loving glances, or try to flirt in a superficial way. Men display their sexual prowess in other ways. Others use sexual energy to gain material goods, position, money, or status. If you use these means, you deprecate your sexual energy and lose the profoundness of this experience at the mental or spiritual level. If you use sex as a means for obtaining something, if you get involved performing "sexual theater," you soon come to a stage where you will entirely forget what it is to be genuine and spontaneous.

७. शंका, भय तथा संशय कामपूर्ति में बाधक है तथा मनोशक्ति से इनका शमन करना चाहिए।

7. **Insecurity, fear, and doubt hinder sexual attraction and fulfillment; such feelings can be conquered through mental control.**

Feelings of insecurity, fear, and doubt may become hindrances in sexual fulfillment in two different ways. First, they may form the general pattern of a person's behavior in all domains of life. Second, they may arise only specifically in relation to one's partner.

A woman's inner doubts, fears, and suspicions diminish even an otherwise beautiful and attractive person. A person who is not physically beautiful may be very appealing and attractive because of qualities like courage and fearlessness, qualities that breed self-assurance and self-confidence.

Fear, insecurity, and doubt are also an obstacle to sexual expression. If you doubt the commitment and sincerity of your partner or fear losing him, you may be unable to immerse yourself fully during sexual congress. Do not encourage such feelings. Truth and honesty should prevail between sexual companions, and any existing doubts should be cleared. Use your mental power, have courage, speak the truth, and be fearless. It is neither good for health nor good for sexual communication to harbor such feelings.

Many women are insecure about losing their charm and beauty with age. They are afraid of getting old, and this fear withers the grace that age would have lent them. Do not attach too much importance to beauty and youth. That is not the only wealth you have. Invest instead in your inner power. Do not live in an imbalanced way. If you are blessed with beauty, do not lose it by dwelling in fear and insecurity. Instead, enhance the power of your mind and live in a holistic way so that you can stay beautiful for a long time.

Around menopause, many women are gripped with the fear that they have come to an end of their youth and have stepped into old age. First, realize that stepping from youth to old age is a very slow phenomenon. Decay is an integral part of the physical body; it commences with birth. Children are happy to grow old. After a few youthful years, adults stop enjoying the process because they attach too much importance to their physical self and do not accept the eternal phenomenon of time. They look at time only from within their one lifespan, but life does not cease with one person. Besides, every period of life unfolds a wealth of new experiences with their own charm and beauty.

Women should not think sexual life diminshes after forty. Feel enriched, rather, with the wisdom and experience you have accumulated in your twenties and thirties. If you feel you've missed something, now is the time to pick up courage to do it. Do not grow old with regrets. The time after forty is the time for realization and reflection. Do not let the fear of old age spoil the most precious years of your life.

८. नित्यता का भाव एक भ्रम है जो मन में नहीं रखना चाहिए।

8. The idea of permanence is illusory; do not even entertain it.

Permanence is a mere illusion. The great epic the *Mahabharata* points out that the most surprising thing in the world is that though hundreds of people die every day, the rest still think they will stay here forever. Direct your mental effort towards attaining this fundamental wisdom: nothing stays forever, and everything is constantly changing. The Hindu tradition goes so far as to say that even the phenomenal world comes to dissolution one day when its cause—the union of the Universal Soul and the Cosmic Substance, the Purusha and the Prakriti—is no longer there.

Feelings such as fear and insecurity arise because we want to believe in our own permanence. Yet life is nothing but the sum total of the changes occurring constantly in this universe. Conception occurs; an embryo grows, is born, goes through childhood, youth, and old age, and ultimately dies. If things did not change, there would be no phenomenal universe. Capturing this basic truth of life enables us to live fearlessly, contented and happier.

६. वर्तमान क्षण में अपने पूरे मनोबल से लीन होने का अभ्यास करना चाहिए।

9. Train yourself to concentrate with all your intensity on the present moment.

Take this sutra in the context of the previous one—that permanence does not exist in this ever-changing universe. With that in mind, learn to dwell in the present moment, and become involved with all energy and force in the task at hand. To master this attitude requires self-discipline, long-term training, and perseverance. Such an outlook to life can bring great intensity to your life; increase your efficiency, productivity, and creativity; and can bring you contentment and peace of mind.

Use this ability to dwell in the present moment at the time of sexual union. Changes are always taking place in sexual communication, behavior, and intensity. Some people keep glorifying the past and pine for "what was." In the process, they make their present relationship worse. Do not linger on what was and, instead, try to make the best of what is.

During sexual union, the senses first express themselves through activity, or rajas; one then steps into tamas for a while, and then to sattva—which gives rise to an experience of momentary bliss. Immerse yourself in that beatitude. The constant practice of singlepointedness of mind and the ability to live in the present can prolong the moment of bliss.

१०. सहभोगी के चुनाव के समय उसकी शारीरिक तथा मानसिक अनुरूपता पर ध्यान देना आवश्यक है।

10. Coordination between physical and mental capacities is essential in choosing a partner.

The physical and mental capacities of two sexual partners should coordinate. One cannot lead a fulfilling life when each aspect is treated as a distinct fragment. Many factors cause attraction between two persons. Companionship and friendship arise from sharing of values, lifestyles, philosophical ideas, hobbies, passions, and so forth. Sexuality is a special kind of sharing which cannot be separated from the other aspects. Sexuality is experienced at physical, mental, and spiritual levels. When two individuals communicate harmoniously, they go through the pains and perils of life together and get tuned to each other. Then, fondness helps them experience sexuality in all its dimensions.

Personal effort can help with physical and mental coordination. But there are limits, especially, when the two individuals are mentally or physically on different ends of the spectrum. Let me take some examples. Suppose you are an artist of repute and the man you have as your partner has no interest in your dancing or painting or singing. His world is limited to the basics of life; he believes that a profession is for earning money, and eating and drinking well and making love on the weekends are enough for him. You are unable to share with him your artistic passion. Despite being good-looking, healthy, and energetic, this kind of man would not be compatible for a profound sexual experience. In fact, a journey within (spiritual experience through sexuality) can help enhance the creativity of an artist.

If you are an adventurous person and like to explore the world, be careful not to pick a kapha-dominated person who goes for a holiday at the same or similar place year after year and orders the same menu again and again. This person will not be able to explore with you the diverse dimensions of sexuality.

Many women live in the illusion that they can change or mold their partners. Without doubt, women have more ability than men to change others because of their high level of sattva. However, influencing others merely to satisfy your ego or have your way is destructive both to you and to your partner. Using the force of your mind towards a desired change may give positive results. But the aim should be selfless, not ego-oriented.

A person who suffers from complexes or who believes in the strict division of work for a man and a woman is also not an appropriate partner to explore the immensity of sexuality. This kind of man will never evoke the eternal female within him. He may have sexual vigor but be unable to satisfy you on the emotional plane. This can become a hindrance in sexual expression, and you will remain at a superficial level of sexual sharing.

The preceding examples are equally valid for men when they are choosing a partner. Men often place more emphasis than women on physical attraction, ignoring the mental realm. Such companionships are hopeless, fated to remain at a very superficial level. The two companions get bored with each other in a few years, and sexuality dies out after a while.

११. काम सम्बन्धों द्वारा बहुदर्शन अनुभूति प्राप्त करने के लिए दोनों सहभोगियों में आदर, सहानुभूति अनुकम्पा तथा सद्भाव होना चाहिए।

11. Respect, sympathy, understanding, and compassion are essential for encompassing broader horizons of sexual experience.

"Broader horizons of sexual experience" means the experience of spirituality through sexuality, a theme treated in Part XI. To have a spiritual experience through sexuality, both partners have to completely transcend their physical self and reach the level of pure consciousness. To do this, they need to be in complete harmony with each other. For harmony, understanding is essential. If two people respect each other and have sympathy for each other, it is easier for them to understand each other's point of view. Neither tries to impose his or her views on the other. They reach a harmonious level through understanding. It is not kindness or pity the two companions need to have for one another. Man and woman are complementary to each other; one is incomplete without the other. Compassion means feeling the pain of the other as your own, with an intensity as if you were yourself the sufferer. When two companions are able to achieve this level of intense feelings for each other, it becomes easier for them to reach the level of oneness during sexual union.

नारी कामसूत्र के सातवें भाग की इति होती है। इसमें मानसिक शक्ति का काम के साथ सम्बन्ध बताया गया है।

This brings to an end Part VII of *The Kamasutra for Women* on the relationship between mental power and sexuality.

PART VIII
Atmosphere, Rituals, and Sexuality

• • •

आठवाँ भाग
वातावरण तथा रीतियों का काम से सम्बन्ध

• • •

Oh lady! Just like a small straw which whirls around the wind, I stir your mind so that you begin to desire me and may not stay away from me. May this woman come to me with a desire for a husband. Desiring her, I may also completely give myself to her. I have come to her with wealth just like a best horse goes to his female counterpart.

—*Atharva Veda*

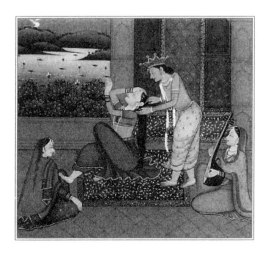

९. सत्त्व और तमस् की अधिकता होने से स्त्रियाँ अपनी काम भावना को मन्द गति एवं सौम्यता से अभिव्यक्त करती हैं।

1. Due to the dominance of sattva and tamas, women are slower and gentler in their sexual expression.

The fundamental nature of women and men is different. Women tend to be shy and hesitant in expressing their feelings and desires, and hesitant in revealing their bodies. A slow and romantic building of the sexual atmosphere invigorates desire and prepares them for profound and intense expression. They need confidence and assurance, and it takes them time to gain momentum in sexual activity.[1]

Women should not deny this part of their being. They should not let themselves be forced into a situation. In recent years, many women have begun to think that their path to freedom lies in being similar to men, and in this process they discard their shyness and hesitancy and assume the quick and direct expression of many men. Some organized groups of women's movements believe that shyness and slow sexual expression are socially imposed, not natural qualities.

We can see this is not true if we observe feminine sexuality in its totality. For example, a woman does not behave like a man at the physical level. A man can reach the limit of his sexual activity rather quickly, with his orgasm, but a woman usually needs more time, more sexual activity. Look at this also at the symbolic, physiological level of egg and sperm: the egg is single, big, copious, a storehouse of nourishment, slow in mobility. Sperms are innumerable, light, fast, and competitive. Sperms travel to the egg. The egg has a tough outer membrane which the sperm must pierce.

Woman's slow, shy sexual behavior is an outward manifestation of her inner sexual nature. Ignoring this basic nature in favor of more direct and aggressive sexual expression only creates an imbalance. If women imbibe more rajas, they will lack sattva and tamas. They will become "like men." Would not such a unisex world be uninteresting and boring?

Women can actually harm themselves in their race to be "equal" to men. An example is that more and more women have taken to smoking during recent years and the rate of lung cancer among them has increased dramatically. Such reactions are counterproductive and abusive.

You should act, not react. Use your creative powers to cure the ills of the society. Men have something you do not have—bigger builds, more physical strength—and you have something they do not have—stability, creative power, intuitive knowledge. There is no reason for a fight—there is too much to appreciate in each other!

२. रजस की अधिकता होने के कारण पुरुष का स्वभाव इससे विपरीत होता है।

2. Men are dominated by rajas, and therefore behave differently from women.

It is important to understand that the degree of this domination varies according to the specific male–female ratio of each person. Men who have a relatively high ratio of the female principle are slower in sexual expression, while men on the other extreme may put off some women with their rapidity and overenthusiasm. In this respect, men and women should act with common sense and wisdom. First try to know yourself, then observe the other objectively.

३. काम में एकलय होने तथा उसके प्रबल अनुभव के लिए प्रारम्भ में धैर्य तथा मंथर गति आवश्यक है।

3. A gentle beginning and patience are essential for harmony and intensity in sexual experience.

The quality of patience is getting lost with the advancement of technology and industrialization. Fast-food culture has crept into sexuality. People have slowly forgotten the meaningful customs and rituals of the past that brought them consciousness, and they have learned to "pass by" life without really living it.

For most young people in the West, togetherness *begins* with sexuality; the slow and steady experience of getting to know each other seems a thing of the past. What has happened to the culture of the serenades? A song such as George Brassens's "The Lovers on the Public Benches" from the early 1950s seems a distant legend. (The song tells of the green benches along the footpaths of a park, and of the young lovers on these benches who hold hands and exchange glances of love and passion and make plans for the future.)

Many rituals which added color to man–woman relationships are slowly becoming extinct. Yet these small gestures, ceremonies, and rituals can bring to us a realization of the intensity of life in human beings.

In India, the ancient tradition of arranged or organized marriages is still followed by a large segment of the society. This means that sexuality begins only after marriage and that companionship is established only in the course of time. In former times, the marriage ceremony used to last for several days, and the ceremony involved many rituals to mentally prepare the couple for sexuality and to romanticize it. Many playful ceremonies were performed during the time immediately after marriage. The couple was not usually allowed to sleep together for some days after the marriage, though customs varied from region to region.

Here is a citation from the *Kamasutra of Vatsyayana* to highlight the traditional views on the subject:

> *For the first three days after their marriage, husband and wife should sleep on the floor and abstain from intercourse. . . . For the next seven days, they should bathe to the sound of music,*

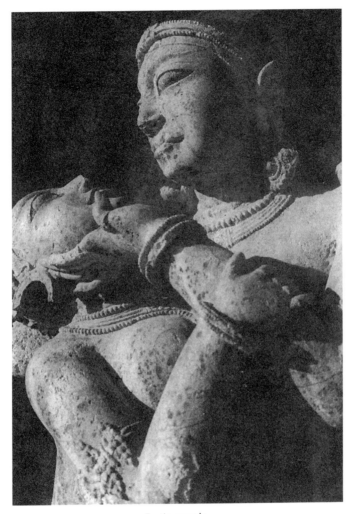

Erotic couple.

adorn themselves, dine together and pay their respects to their
relatives and to the other people who attended their wedding. . . .
On the evening of the tenth day, the husband should speak gently
to his wife to give her confidence. He should refrain from inter-
course until he has won over his bride's confidence, as women,
being gentle by nature, prefer to be won over gently. If a woman
is roughly handled by a man whom she scarcely knows, she may

come to hate sexuality and to hate the whole male sex. Or, she may detest her husband in particular, and then will turn to another man.[2]

It is interesting to note how modernization has transformed the system of arranged marriages. The marriage ceremony is mostly a short one these days, especially in the cities. The ceremonious preparations, which had deep physiological and psychological importance, are rapidly vanishing. Both men and women, often unable to meet the expectations of one another, suffer. With a rather nervous and fearful attitude, many women let themselves be subjected to sex rather than participating actively and enjoying it. The men, who lack self-confidence, develop problems with their sexuality. In this process, they become aggressive in order to prove their "manliness." From Punjab, the most modernized of all the Indian states, we know of some ridiculous cases where a woman left her husband after the first night of the marriage, declaring him impotent.

Whether partners choose each other or come together as a result of familial arrangements, rituals and ceremonies can help to harmonize the sexual energy within, and help make it a stable flame rather than a spark that ignites quickly and vanishes. Both men and women need patience and indulgence with each other. A rapid pace, whether at the beginning of a relationship or during sexual interaction, does not lead to a complete sexual experience.

४. उपयुक्त वातावरण से लक्ष्य प्राप्ति में सरलता होती है।

4. An appropriate atmosphere further enhances sexual intensity.

The priority of creating a suitable environment and atmosphere for important activities in our lives is fast diminishing. The small ceremonies and rituals from all different cultures that have traditionally helped people slide from one activity to another have been forgotten. We never learn complete expression of the senses, or how to turn momentary bliss into a profound experience of pure consciousness.

We seem to be evolving into a "switch on/switch off" culture. Yet advancements in technology do not constitute a culture. People keep a television in their bedrooms. Immediately after the sports match or horror film, they want the "joy of sex." Such rapidity precludes the possibility of physical communication that is truly different, personal, and profound. Sexuality ends up as just another superficial pleasure of life.

Keep your bedroom free of television. Decorate it in light and soft colors, and do not clutter it with too many things. Soft music and a few attractive pictures are enough. Keep it properly ventilated and mildly perfumed.

Some women believe that wearing sexy, transparent night dresses can help build an atmosphere. Such sexual excitement is momentary. The idea is not to "vomit out" your sexual desire and be done with it, but to find expression of all the senses, to intensify sensuality.

CONCENTRATION EXERCISE

Here's a simple example for a couple who may want to build up atmosphere and attain stillness of mind:

Wear loose white clothes and sit down in front of each other. Close your eyes and concentrate on your power of hearing. Visualize the form of your ears. Take a deep breath and hold it inside by closing both nostrils. Slowly let the air out.

Now concentrate on the sense of touch by visualizing your whole body. After that, concentrate on your sense of sight by visualizing your eyes. Then concentrate on the sense of taste, think about your tongue, and visualize it inside your mouth. Do the same with the sense of smell by concentrating on your nose.

After having concentrated on all your five senses, concentrate on the middle of your eyebrows and take three vital breaths. After this short ceremony, open your eyes and look at each other. Close your eyes again and concentrate on the five senses of your partner with five vital breaths. After this ceremony, slowly approach each other.

---

५. प्राकृतिक दृश्यों तथा अन्य आनन्दवर्धक अनुभवों से स्त्री विश्वस्त तथा निःशंक हो जाती है तथा काम भाव प्रबल रूप से प्रकट करती है।

5. Observing nature and sharing pleasurable experiences brings confidence and trust to a woman and can make her sexual expression intense.

The sharing of the small pleasures of life provides the woman a sense of togetherness and gives her confidence and faith in her companion. Watching the evening sky together, taking a walk, and going near a water source are some simple things a couple can do easily. A man and a woman who come home from their respective jobs, or a man coming from work and a woman busy with children at home need to make an effort to get out of their routine and refresh their companionship.

६. इससे उसका रचनात्मक पक्ष प्रोत्साहित होता है तथा वह क्रियाशील और कुशल हो जाती है।

6. Feelings of companionship evoke a woman's creative dimension: she becomes active and innovative.

Feelings of companionship give rise to confidence and faith in a woman and emphasize the sattva, which is responsible for her creativity. Her creative aspect unfolds itself in sexuality, and she becomes innovative and active. At this stage her doubts and hesitations vanish as she begins the journey into a profound realm, from which she is able to express herself completely. Spontaneously she discovers new ways of expression and communication and uncovers the hidden treasures of pleasure and exhilaration. Because of sattva, her concentration and energy increase.

७. अपने रचनात्मक भावोदय के कारण वह पुरुष का सत्त्व उत्तेजित करती है जिससे उसकी ग्रहण शक्ति बढ़ती है।

7. Her creative dimension also evokes sattva in the man, which increases his power of retention.

The innovative dimension of a woman during sexual communication evokes sattva in her companion. In response to her unhindered sexual expression, his sexual activity increases, and due to enhanced sattva, his power to prolong the sexual act also increases. It all works in a sequence of action and response. This is why an appropriate beginning is so important.

८. इससे स्त्री की भावना और भी प्रबल हो जाती है तथा उसकी प्रभूत शक्ति प्रवाहित होने लगती है ।

8. His prolonged activity further intensifies her experience, leading to a smooth flow of abundant sexual energy.

When the man is able to prolong his sexual activity, the woman's sexual experience intensifies in response. In fact, it is at this time that her sexual energy flows most abundantly. This is the time of the most intense experience for a woman, when each part of her body is invigorated and she is about to reach a state when she transcends her senses. Woman must realize that to reach this experience of complete fulfillment requires effort and coordination from both partners.

९. विविध रीतियों से यह अनुभूति दीर्घकालिक की जा सकती है।

9. Ritualistic practices can prolong and intensify sexual experience.

Sutra 4 described one simple ritual for concentrating the mind. Here I will go into the more technical details of the body and subtle energy, a concept that has been very well elaborated in the ritualistic Tantric tradition.

Like the rest of the cosmos, the body is made of five elements, as noted earlier. These elements give rise to the three humors, which are responsible for the physical and mental functions of the body. All of this remains at the material level. However, the five elements are also represented symbolically at the subtle level in different parts of the body: earth, between feet and knees; water, between knees and anus; fire, between anus and solar plexus; air, between solar plexus and eyebrows; and ether, between eyebrows and the top of the head.

Within the material body, the subtle body is made up of a network of channels through which the prana circulates. This subtle energy is everywhere and in each part of our body, but it also has three principal channels which cross each other at six points. These confluent points of energy are called chakras.

The six chakras represent the five senses and the mind, and the seventh chakra represents the state of pure consciousness obtained by transcending all sensuality. This state consists of the oneness of the soul with the cosmic energy. The three principal energy channels originate from the level of the anus, where the dormant power, or *kundalini*, lies. Symbolically, kundalini is represented in the coiled form, which is also the literal meaning of this word. Once

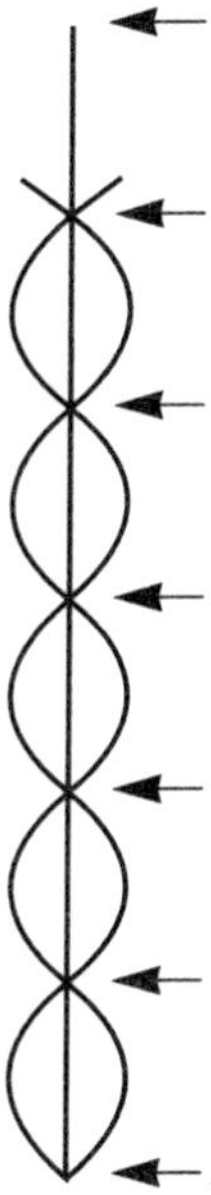

Location in the Body	Name	Symbolic Sound: Mantra	Element	Vital Activity
Top of the head	Sahasrara	Beyond all sounds; denotes the Universal Soul	Universal Soul	Beyond all activities
Between eyebrows	Ajna	OM	Mind	Mental functions
Throat	Vishuddha	Ham	Ether	Hearing
Plexus	Anahata	Yam	Air	Touch
Navel	Manipura	Ram	Fire	Sight
Genitals	Svadhishthana	Vam	Water	Taste
Anus	Muladhara	Lam	Earth	Smell

Figure 28   A diagrammatic representation of the three principal channels of the subtle body and location of the concentric energy points, or chakras. The name, symbolic sound (mantra), corresponding element, and vital activity of each chakra is also given.

you have achieved mastery in pranayama, you can, with power of concentration and singlepointedness of mind, evoke this dormant energy. However, it is not an easy task. It requires perseverance and persistence over a long period of time.

Figure 28 shows the details of the seven chakras, their names, their location in the body, their symbolic sounds, or mantras, their corresponding elements, and their vital activity. By repeating the mantra of each chakra, you can slowly increase your power of concentration and develop singlepointedness. This evokes the dormant power of kundalini, increases the energy level in the body, and enhances sexual capability, expression, and fulfillment. For more details on the subject, you may refer to other books on Tantra.[3] However, Tantric concepts are often used very superficially in the West, as a salable commodity in the form of books, seminars, and workshops. Be careful to consult books from a reliable authority, as many recent books offer mostly misleading information.

You must realize that a chakra's influence is not limited to only a small point where the three principal channels cross. From this given point, it encircles the whole body at its level. The lowest chakra represents the heaviest element—the earth—and as they ascend, they represent ever lighter elements. The fifth chakra represents the cosmic element ether. The sixth chakra symbolizes the mind. The seventh chakra is above the head; it represents Absolute Energy.

For our purposes, the most important chakras are the first and the fourth. The first chakra (*muladhara*) represents the *linga* (the male sexual organ) inside the *yoni* (the female sexual organ) (Fig. 29). The fourth chakra (*anahata*) symbolizes the ultimate union and fulfillment of the male and female principles (see Part II). This

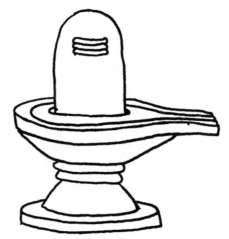

Figure 29   Shivalinga in the Yoni pedestal.

chakra represents union at the cosmic level, while the first chakra represents sexual union.

१०. योग की विधियों से कुण्डलिनी शक्ति भी जागृत की जा सकती है।

10. The dormant energy of kundalini can be evoked with yogic practices.

The dormant power of the kundalini can be evoked through the methods of pranayama and singlepointedness of the mind. A long practice of concentrating on each chakra leads to a transcending of the physical plane. As the kundalini traverses the various chakras in an upward direction, you begin to sense its deeper power.

SINGLEPOINTEDNESS OF THE MIND THROUGH PRANAYAMA

The path to singlepointedness[4] of the mind becomes an easier one with the help of pranayama practices, as described in Part VI. During these practices, the mind concentrates on the inhalation and exhalation of the vital air, and all other activities are silenced in the process. Singlepointedness of the mind is to bring the mind to this state of stillness when all activity ceases. Constant practice is required to reach this aim.

The first, simple step is to begin concentrating upon one of the objects of your senses. For example, inhale some pleasant-smelling thing, and while you hold the vital air inside you, concentrate your mind completely on this particular smell.

After doing that a few times, try to concentrate on the same smell, but in the abstract, without having it in front of you. Recall it. Assimilate it completely within yourself. In this process, the mind gets immersed in, and evenutaly dwells exclusively on this experience.

Repeated practice will give you the capacity to prolong this sensing at will. Do the same for the other senses. Concentrate on some sound, visual object, taste, or tactile sensation. Your aim at the beginning is to concentrate upon the whole sensuous experience, but later you should try to forget the medium and dwell only on the experience.

For example, if you concentrate on a visual object, you may in the beginning look at it; later you will close your eyes, and only the appearance of the object should remain in your mind. After a while, even the appearance should not remain—only the essence of the object should be there. In this state, the rationale for the name, form, and so on disappears.

The next step is to practice concentrating upon each of the five elements. With each vital breath, concentrate on one quality of that particular element. For example, if you are concentrating on air, think of it in various forms such as movement, stillness, omnipresence, and life-giving force. After you have thought of all its qualities, dwell on only its elemental form. Do the same for the other four elements. It is better to practice concentrating on each element regularly for several weeks.

Once you've trained the mind to dwell upon a single object, you may begin to concentrate on each chakra one by one. Begin from the lowest one, the muladhara chakra. Guide your prana energy there. Concentrate your mind on the location of this chakra. It represents the element earth in your body. Do this practice every day for a month. If you have trouble concentrating, initiate the concentration by repeating the mantra "Lam," which symbolizes this energy point. When you get lost in the sound, repeat the mantra only in your thoughts. Slowly stop even the sound. The only thing remaining should be that particular energy point.

Concentrate on each chakra every month, and eventually you will revitalize your whole body and mind. As mentioned in the preceding sutra, the first and the fourth chakras represent, respectively, sexual and cosmic union. By concentrating on these energy points, you can achieve any specific aim you have in mind or solve any related physical, mental, or spiritual problem. First, however, you have to have mastered pranayama and continued regular concentration practice for seven months on each chakra. Superficially repeating the mantra for each chakra will not suffice.

Do not begin concentration practices with the aim of achieving something at the sexual level, although this will happen spontaneously. Practice the mantra for each chakra regularly every day for a few minutes in the mornings and evenings. Continue this for several months, proceeding upwards slowly. This practice will not only enrich your sexual experience but also improve your quality of life as you develop extraordinary sensitivity and intuition. The concentration practices on the chakras can help heal any ailment related to that particular sense organ.

११. मनुष्य की अथाह सृजन शक्ति के प्रयोग से सहभोगियों को अपनी व्यक्तिगत रीतियों का निर्माण करना चाहिए।

11. Couples should use their creative power to formulate their own personal rituals.

The kind of disciplined routine that we have to live in most of the time can make life very mechanical and boring. Humans need to experience something new, different, adventurous, and exciting.

Constant overhauling and maintenance of body, mind, and behavior are required to avoid getting into a rut. Wise persons should consciously make efforts to rejuvenate themselves and change according to place and time. Human beings are endowed with the discretion and intellect to bring new life to their sexual expression.

Invent new ways and methods, and do diverse things. Certain things can be learned from outside sources, but remember the immense source of knowledge hidden within. Do not let your inner light be covered with the dust gathered from old routines. Renew yourself.

नारी कामसूत्र के आठवें भाग की यहां इति होती है।
इसमें वातावरण तथा रीतियों का काम
से सम्बन्ध बताया गया है।

This brings to an end Part VIII of *The Kamasutra for Women*, explaining the importance of atmosphere and rituals for sexual expression.

PART IX
*R*hythm and *V*ariety in *S*exuality

. . .

नवाँ भाग
काम में विविधता तथा लय

. . .

Women have eight times more sexual energy than men.
—*Canakya, Vatsyayana, and many others*

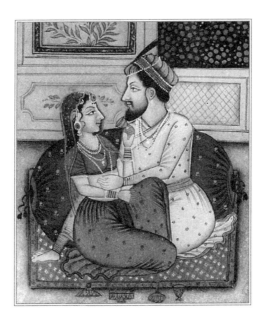

१. सभी इन्द्रियों की तृप्ति एवं काम-सुख के लिए, स्त्री और पुरुष दोनों की साधना तथा श्रम आवश्यक है।

1. Complete sensuous fulfillment and sexual satisfaction require a joint effort and dedication of both partners.

Sexual fulfillment is like any other success in life. Concentration, effort, and devotion are needed to make the sexual act a unique experience every time. Some people may argue that sexuality, being a natural urge, hardly requires conscious effort. But human beings differ from animals in their sexuality.

२. यद्यपि कामेच्छा तथा काम-सुख स्वाभाविक हैं किन्तु मनुष्य अपनी बुद्धि और बल से इसमें वृद्धि या ह्रास कर सकता है।

2. Although the desire for sexuality and the pleasure resulting from the act are innate, human beings are capable of destroying or intensifying it with their intellect and power of discretion.

Human beings are capable of enhancing, diminishing, or ruining the innate character of their sensuality. We can enhance it by assimilating knowledge transferred from one generation to the next, through art and writing. However, the power of discretion and intellect may also become a hindrance in expressing sexuality freely. Values, rules, and superstitions may get in the way. In a flexible and tolerant society, human variations are easily accepted, but in societies with strict social norms, people are expected to behave according to certain set patterns. The denial of the eternal feminine principle in the man and of the masculine principle in the woman then gives rise to multiple sexual problems, as well as to social evils.

Society is made up of the collective strength of us all. We must not hesitate to change society's values when need be. In recent years, we realized that a polluted environment, disease, and the side effects of chemical drugs and adulterated foods are leading humanity towards destruction. Only a turn towards the ancient holistic way of life will allow us to regain the lost equilibrium in our societies, as well as in our personal lives.

Although sexuality is a natural urge, it is under assault from our fragmented way of living, as are other natural human needs and urges. Sleep is a natural urge, but many people take drugs in order

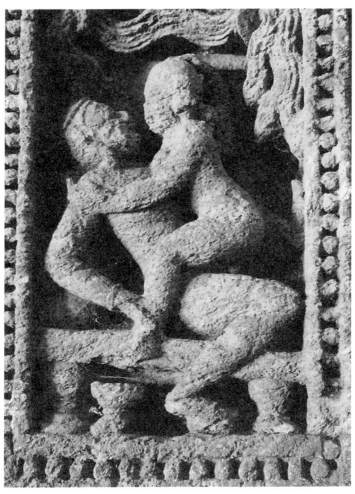

Erotic couple.

to sleep. Digestion is a natural process, but millions today cannot digest their food properly. What is not needed by the body should be excreted every day, but how many in this world are suffering from constipation? We must bring back the natural rhythm of our lives.

ENHANCING VAGINAL SECRETION

Many women suffer from a lack of vaginal secretion during sexual activity. This may be due to diverse reasons. Vaginal infections or inflammations may hinder the timely mucous secretion. This, however, will be accompanied by some other pathological symptoms, and you should cure this problem by taking an appropriate treatment.

Lack of vaginal secretion may also be due to psychological reasons like fear, anxiety, loss of interest in one's partner, or a desire for some other man. You should try to find the reasons in your case and go to the root of the problem to find out the cause of this ill effect.

According to ancient Indian literature on sexuality, the site of vaginal secretion, or *kama jal* ("sexual water"), is the moon channel (the left of the three principal channels running along the spine). Thus, women suffering from this ailment should do purification of the channels by laying emphasis especially on the moon channel. While doing this practice, they should concentrate on their vagina and direct the prana energy there.

Many women have problems with vaginal secretion during sexual activity. Due to one reason or another, their vagina remains "dry," despite the sexual activity. You may direct all the energy of the sexual impulse to revitalize your vaginal cells and rejuvenate them. You will realize that this force is so strong that you may feel its effect immediately.

In addition to all this, you may want to try the following treatments:

1. Take a soft vegetable like a zucchini, peel it, and cut a piece. Dip the piece in honey and insert it into the vagina for a while.

Do not overuse this honey method, since it can have an astringent effect.

2. Mix milk skin with honey and licorice powder and apply to the vaginal walls. A mixture of 1/4 teaspoon each of licorice, honey, and milk skin will make an effective preparation. To get the milk skin, boil a quantity of milk for about ten minutes, cool it, and place it in the refrigerator for a few hours. The thin film which appears on top is milk skin. Natural or raw milk will produce a thicker layer than the homogenized variety.

3. A massage of your palms and soles by your partner can also help solve the problem.

---

३. सब सुखों में काम सुख को सर्वोपरि मानकर तथा कल्पना से ही भोग कर व्यर्थ नहीं करना चाहिए।

3. Do not waste sexual energy by dwelling on the thought of future sexual pleasure and its immensity.

Both partners need to retain their energy if they are to bring rhythm and variety to the sexual act. Many people fantasize too much about a coming sexual experience, imagining it the greatest of all pleasures. No doubt sexual experience is one of the greatest gifts of nature. To enjoy this bliss, it's best not to fire your sexual energy with wild imagination even beforehand. Many people expect too much out of sexual interaction and are disappointed with their introduction to the real thing. All our lives we have to make an effort to achieve success in our projects; sexuality is not an exception.

There is another reason for this disappointment. Many people believe that the only real sexuality is sexual intercourse, and because such intercourse is taboo in their situation, they keep postponing it, while indulging in all manner of other sexual activities. Intercourse is then kept for some special, future occasion. I have found this behavior among young people, of course, before their first sexual experience, but also among partners who have a bad conscience about maintaining a sexual relationship outside their regular couple relationship. To save themselves from guilt, they communicate with their partners sexually at many levels except for intercourse. Such people often build up expectations about their partner—yet such compartmentalized living inevitably leads to disappointment. Do not create for yourself such boundaries and lines, and do not live in a hypocritical world of your own. Such behavior hinders your spontaneity, harms your sexual life in general, and may have a long-lasting bad effect on you.

Another category of people build a pile of expectations for a particular person, and when at last, after waiting too long for this "extraordinary" person to agree, they are disenchanted with their sexual pleasure.

Men or women who have a rather late sexual awakening, due to shyness or some other reason, may also suffer excessive fantasizing.

CHANNELING SEXUAL ENERGY TO PRESERVE IT

Sexual energy is very powerful, and you should not suppress or waste it. It should be channeled with the right methods. If you try to suppress it, it may acquire volcanic dimensions and may erupt in the form of mental or physical ailments or abnormal sexual behavior.

It is relatively easier to enhance the sexual expression than to preserve or channel the sexual energy. These two can be compared to making a canal for the flow of the water from a river and making a dam. Channeling sexual energy requires a mastery of concentration skills. When the mind is still, it gets spiritual energy and is able to direct and control physical and mental activities.

If you are impelled very forcefully by a sexual urge at a wrong time, learn to retain this force with the following method. Do not get discouraged if you do not succeed the first time. Just keep practicing it with a determined mind and persistence in achieving your aim.

Concentrate on your abdominal region, which is the seat of sexual impulse and its release, at the moment you are impelled by this force. Breathe in smoothly and profoundly. At the time you are letting the vital air enter within yourself, pull up with force the energy from the pelvic region towards the solar plexus. Exhale smoothly. Try this a few times. You will be relieved of the force of sexual impulse. You may have a feeling of heat in your body. You will experience complete stillness. The state of excitement will turn into peace and well-being. The sexual energy is not lost but transformed and preserved.

Sexual energy is also preserved by the rapid breathing method described in step 4 of the pranayama practices (see Part VI, Sutra 10). Concentrate on the impelling force which is produced by the sexual impulse, and begin rapid breathing in such a way as if you are pulling this force up towards your head. This may give you a feeling like you are actually undergoing sexual experience. Afterwards, you will have a feeling of satisfaction and well-being. Rest for a few moments after this, as it is a little tiring due to rapid breathing, as compared to the slower breathing in of vital air as just described.

---

४. काम में लय तथा विविधता लाने के लिए शारीरिक तथा मानसिक शक्ति बढ़ाने के पूर्व वर्णित उपायों का प्रयोग करना चाहिए।

4. Use the mind- and body-strengthening methods previously described to bring rhythm and variety to your sexuality.

You cannot vary your body posture and movements unless you are able to master your body and mind. If your general energy level is low or you are extremely fragile, you will not be able to engage in prolonged sexual congress. With a stiff body, you cannot assume many different postures. Without concentrating your mind, you cannot be creative or prolong your sexual interaction and enhance your sexual vigor.

५. कुछे लोग भ्रमवश यह सोचते हैं कि कामोत्तजना शरीर के कुछ विशेष अंगों तक ही सीमित है।

5. Sexual excitation is not limited to only certain parts of the body.

With some variation, all parts of the body are sexually excitable. However, a continuous period of extreme excitement during sexual congress may render the highly excitable parts relatively less so during the contact. Therefore, a couple should explore and discover different parts of the body. Do this by actively using all parts of your body, from different angles. Explore, for example, the different parts of the sole of the foot, the spaces between the toes, the spaces between the fingers of the hands, all parts of the palm, all places near the joints, and so forth. The tactile sensation should be fully developed through effort and practice. It should have its complete expression, and it should also help to excite the other senses, and vice versa. The tactile sensation is also related to the other four senses, and these five normally work in cooperation with each other during sexual communication.

Your sense of touch can also be excited by slow and deep breathing. Practice of pranayama before sexual congress enhances concentration and the intuitive power of the mind.

People often get bored with each other sexually because they do not use their intellect and physical abilities in their sexual communication. They neither explore themselves nor others, and instead simply look for new excitement in another person. But the new also becomes routine. Knowingly or unknowingly, too many

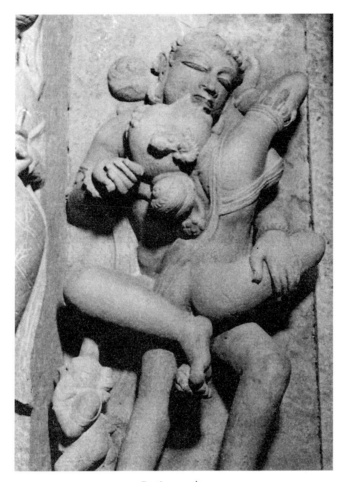

Erotic couple.

people treat sexuality like driving a car. It is very exciting in the beginning when you're learning to drive, but after a while, it becomes second nature and you don't have to think much. It may be exciting at first to change the cars, to buy a faster or a more elegant looking one, but this too becomes routine after a while. If sexuality becomes a routine, you will be as disappointed with several partners as with one. If you live in a fragmented way, treat your body like a machine, and compartmentalize your life, you obviously cannot be very adventurous in exploring the sexual potential within you and your partner. You can tap the vast sexual energy within only by learning to live with the cosmic rhythm.

६. योगाभ्यास आदि से विभिन्न अंगों को क्रियाशील बनाना चाहिए तथा संभोग के समय इनका उपयोग करना चाहिए।

6. Revitalize the different parts of the body through yogic practices and benefit from them during sexual union.

You can revitalize internal and external parts of the body through the special slow movements I have described previously. It is not necessary or possible to practice all these methods every day, but fifteen minutes a day of alternating with various yogic postures should not be a problem. After your body is flexible enough, you may want to learn a set of twelve yogic exercises called Salutation to the Sun.[1] Performing these twelve times every day will not take more than twelve minutes and will invigorate your whole body. Some yogic postures and movements described in Part VI are especially beneficial for making a variety of sexual postures.

Many other ancient methods from China and Japan can bring about flexibility and body awareness. Such athletic efforts as gymnastics, jogging, and running are usually worthless in awakening the body's dormant potentials, since they treat the body as distinct from the mind and not integrated with it. Such exercise may even cause vata imbalance in the body, leading to stiffness, dry skin, and lack of sexual secretions.

७. काम-ज्ञान केवल पुस्तकों से एवं तर्क से नहीं प्राप्त किया जा सकता।

7. Sexual wisdom cannot be obtained merely from books or through argumentative knowledge.

In ancient times, one imbibed wisdom from the elders, from experience, from observation of nature, and from the rituals and ceremonies that accompanied daily living. Texts transmitted wisdom of a teacher or wise person of the community. Life still goes on this way in various tribal and ethnic societies of the world, but in our modern way of living, life has changed considerably. People have become individualistic, the joint or extended family system has broken down, and even the nuclear family is suffering.

These days, books are published on nearly everything. When I was in the United States, I began to learn ice skating. A friend presented me a book on the subject. For us Indians, it is always a matter of great surprise when an average Western woman takes out a recipe book to cook. In recent years, some "modern" women in Delhi and Bombay have started to do the same.

If you adhere strictly to the techniques learned only from books, you risk losing your spontaneity and spirit of innovation. Books which describe mere techniques can also be dangerous if they provide knowledge without the wisdom to use it. Let me give as an example a book on postures to increase sexual pleasure. It may tell you, say, to put your right leg on the shoulder of your male partner while the two of you are engaged in sexual union. Without appropriate preparation to make your joints flexible, attempting such a posture will result in nothing but physical torture—and those suffering from constipation will have it even worse! Such books do not take into consideration your body and mind in totality, and they are simply meant to be sensational.

This is an extreme example, and there are better books. But even if a book is full of wisdom, you cannot become wise by merely reading it. Sexual wisdom is obtained by living a holistic way, by developing your physical and mental strength, by evoking your inner power, and by learning from experience. When you are in harmony within yourself and with your surroundings, you will spontaneously discover the immense pleasures nature has provided us, among which is sexuality.

Select your books wisely and don't get fascinated by pictures or overblown language. It's easy to get trapped by books that make everything in life simple and prescribe methods for "rediscovering your lost pleasures in ten days." Such appeals are simply an extension of the modern world's consumerism, in which everything is short-lived.

You must realize that real wisdom is not space and time bound. The *Yoga Sutra of Patanjali*, the principles of Ayurveda, and the *Kamasutra of Vatsyayana* are examples of the immense sources of wisdom from the ancient world. After thousands of years these books are still published in the different languages of the world, and the wisdom described in them is still as valid for humanity now as it was then. The books you select should not be based merely on the personal experience of the author but should take into account the large variability in human beings and the expanses of space and time.

Argumentative knowledge is like books. You may attend lectures, workshops, or seminars and take part in endless discussions, but to attain true wisdom, you must use the power of discretion and the intuitive knowledge within. Each situation is unique and requires the real wisdom that can be gained only from such internal questioning.

८. काम में विविधता के अनुभव के लिए नये ढंग तथा उपाय अपनाने आवश्यक हैं।

8. Develop new ways and techniques to experience different facets of sexuality.

Variety in experiencing the different facets of sexuality is helpful not only for the sake of experiencing a complete sensuous expression, but it can also help ensure social stability and safeguard the family structure.

Partners need friendship, faith, and respect for each other if they are to truly savor the diverse facets of sexuality, as well as good health, sexual vigor, energy, and a holistic attitude and way of living. We have already discussed several methods to enhance sexual expression. Now, let us see how to bring variability to the sexual union itself.

Altering movement is essential for variability and change of rhythm in sexual experience. Women should play a vigorous role in this respect and not think they can find enjoyment only when a man is energetic and forceful. Women can never find total sensuous expression unless they participate equally with energy and vigor. There should be times for the man to be still and the woman active. She should vary her movements, for example, up and down with various gradations (Fig. 30). It is important to learn various ways of making spiral movements that go up and down, as well as

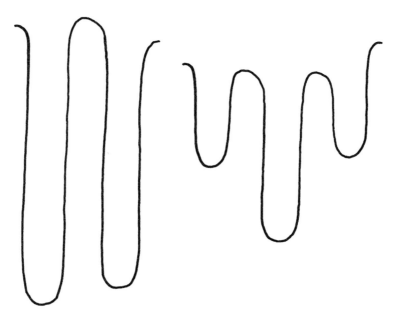

Figure 30   Up-and-down sexual movements are made by altering the depth each time.

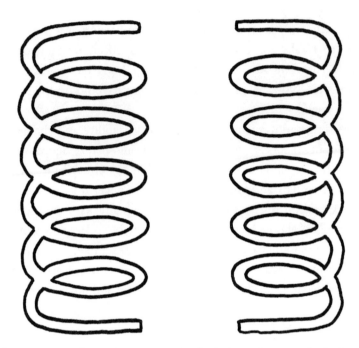

Figure 31   Spiral sexual movements in clockwise and counterclockwise directions.

clockwise and counterclockwise (Fig. 31) Snakelike movements are also very important (Fig. 32). For all these movements, you will need to have a flexible spine.

You may also learn to move in enclosed concentric circles, from the inner to the outer, and then from the outer to the inner (Fig. 33). The same circles can also be made by going upwards and downwards (Fig. 34).

Vary any one type of movement by accelerating and decelerating your speed, then try to switch several times from fast to slow and slow to fast.

Do not think this description is a lesson to be remembered and followed: these are only ideas or suggestions to be slowly assimilated. Practice, experiment, innovate, and create on your own.

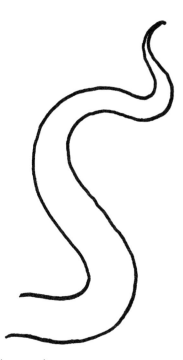

Figure 32   Snakelike sexual movements.

All these movements can be made in different postures; the variability of posture itself depends upon the flexibility of your bodies. However, nearly every couple uses some simple postures which do not need much description. Some examples: the man on his back with the woman sitting upon him; both sitting, sometimes in yoga postures such as lotus or rock; the woman standing, bent, with the man behind her; both lying sideways, with bent knees; the woman on her stomach, with the man on top behind her.

In some conservative societies, a man may find it insulting when a woman moves on him while he lies still. I doubt that any women belonging to these circles will get an opportunity to read this book, but if so, let me say that with love and effort, women can change this attitude. Of course, it will take a very long time to change such societies entirely.

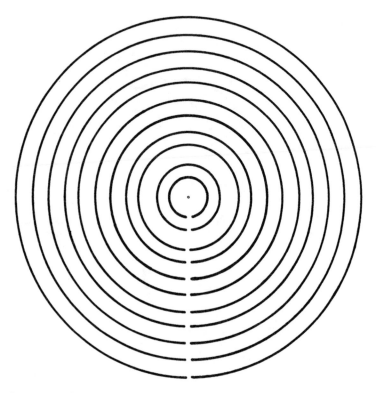

Figure 33 The circular movements involve making concentric circles, from smaller to gradually bigger and then in the reverse. Note that these movements are different from the spiral movements. Here, the smaller circle does not end up in the bigger; rather, there is a small pause after each circle and then an outer (or inner) circle is made afresh.

६. स्त्री और पुरुष द्वारा लम्बे समय तक किये गये पारस्परिक सहयोग एवं प्रयत्न से ही काम का सम्पूर्ण अनुभव होता है तथा काम ज्ञान प्राप्त होता है।

9. A multidimensional joint effort over a period of time leads to sexual experience and wisdom.

If both partners make a serious effort over a long period of time, they will find wholesome sexual experience and sexual wis-

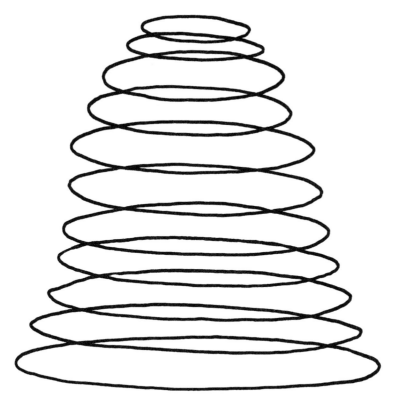

Figure 34   Circles are made by simultaneously varying the depth and the circumference.

dom. A wholesome sexual experience is one in which the senses find their unhindered expression and an intense awakening occurs which is free from the worries of the past and future, provides exhilaration, and leads to beatitude and expansiveness.

१०. इसके लिए सहज स्वाभाविक होना आवश्यक है।

10. Spontaneity is an essential part of sexual wisdom.

Sexuality is a natural phenomenon. In the cosmos, all is connected and everything works in a rhythm. There is variation, yet harmony. Whether for good health or for wholesome sexual experience, we have to be in tune with the cosmic orchestra. Calculated, mechanical moves never lead to fulfillment. A narrow vision and conservative attitude hinder human spontaneity and creativity. These days, too much emphasis on sex education for children can ruin the spontaneity: instead of slowly discovering the mysterious world of sex themselves, children are too often taught sex as an educational subject.

Telling yourself again and again, "Take it easy, be spontaneous," will only make you more stiff, not spontaneous. There is a posture called the dead body posture in yoga. If I tell people to lie down, close their eyes, loosen up, feel heaviness in their bodies, and so on, they end up more tense. They try it at a rational level, and some even frown. Instead, I devise many playful methods to bring them to a state of relaxation—people relax only if they forget they have to relax. Spontaneity in sexual expression cannot be separated from expression in general.

११. काम में सहज स्वाभाविकता तभी आती है जब बाकी जीवन में भी ऐसा ही हो।

11. Spontaneity in sexuality comes only from spontaneity in life itself.

The universe is an interconnected and interrelated vastness, of which you are one part. Understand and follow this basic unity, and have faith in your creativity. You do not learn to be spontaneous by attending seminars or joining cults. I have often seen people carrying this banner: "Just be yourself, just learn to be." But you do not *learn* to be yourself. True being, true living, is not something to be learned, but a realization.

If you observe nature silently in solitude; listen to chirping birds, waterfalls, the sea, and the wind; and observe the strength and awesomeness of the high mountains, the wonder of a tiny seedling which hides the tremendous potential for making a mighty tree, and the variety of colors and forms in this fascinating universe, you will spontaneously realize that you too are a dancer in the cosmic ballet.

नारी कामसूत्र के नवें भाग की यहां इति होती है। इसमें काम में विविधता तथा लय का वर्णन किया गया है।

This brings to an end Part IX of *The Kamasutra for Women*, on rhythm and variety in sexual practice.

PART X
Rejuvenation and Aphrodisiacs

. . .

दसवाँ भाग
कायाकल्प तथा बाजीकरण विधियाँ

. . .

There is no greater aphrodisiac for a woman than a clean,
well-groomed, tenderhearted, and attentive man with a loving
and melodious voice.

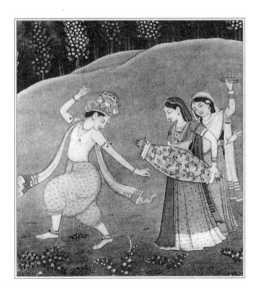

९. विश्व में प्रत्येक वस्तु परिवर्तनशील है तथा मनुष्य का शरीर काल से प्रतिबद्ध है।

1. Everything in the universe is constantly changing, and the human body is bound to time.

While our physical self is bound to time, our soul, the cause of consciousness, is eternal. The body is made of the five elements which constantly transform and reorganize themselves, and in this transformation we pass through the various stages of life, such as childhood, youth, and old age. Nothing is without reason; everything moves towards a goal. During the time between birth and death called an individual's lifespan, a slow and constant decay leads ultimately to death. For a particular person, death may end life, but life continues—the dying makes place for the newborn.

Sexuality is the basis of this cycle of life and death. In the great Indian cosmogonic hymn the *Rig Veda*, it is said that *Kama* was the first step at the beginning of the creation of the universe.[1] The French Indologist Alain Daniélou sums up these philosophical thoughts as follows:

> *The lord of sleep (Shiva), who is the principle of disintegration*
> *(tamas), the source of an ever expanding (disintegrating)*
> *universe, is the principle of time, the destroyer, and at the same*
> *time the embodiment of experience, enjoyment, whose symbol is*
> *the fount of life, the source of pleasure, the phallus (linga).*[2]

Beyond the cycle of birth and death that souls undergo is a cosmic cycle in which all is dissolved into primordial matter, from which everything begins yet again.

The cyclic notion of rebirth and its relation to sexuality is depicted in the *Yogatattva Upanishad* as follows:

> *It is happy, the child that sucks*
> *at its mother's breast;*

it is the same breast it fed from in a former life!
The husband takes his pleasure in his wife's belly;
it was in that same belly he was conceived in the past!
He who was the father, is today the son,
and that son, when tomorrow comes,
will be a father in his turn.[3]

२. बुद्धिमान व्यक्ति को सुखी जीवन के लिए विधिपूर्वक कायाकल्प करना चाहिए।

2. A wise person takes rejuvenating measures to enhance the quality of life.

I use the word *rejuvenation* here in the sense of maintaining and invigorating one's body (the body in the present context also includes mind) to restore and enhance vitality and energy.

In Ayurveda, rejuvenation is a complete therapy that does not consist only of some drugs, and it is prescribed for the sick and convalescing, as well as for healthy persons. Increasing the general energy level of the body helps the sick to recover, and in the healthy it enhances vigor and beauty and works to prevent illness. The methods of rejuvenation vary according to age and condition, and they act on three different levels. First, they act on digestion to increase the assimilation of nutrients. Second, they supplement the diet with invigorating elements. Third, they cleanse open energy channels to enhance the flow of energy in the whole body. Such methods bring harmony between the physical functions of the body and the subtle energy at the level of the chakras.

All of us realize that things decay faster if we do not maintain them. Unpolished wood or iron without paint, exposed to excessive sun or water, will decay very fast. A tea or coffee pot, if not cleaned properly, will change its color forever. Even a glass which we may use only to drink water needs daily cleaning. Yet most people do not think that their internal body organs also need a regu-

lar cleaning and revitalization, or that their mind, constantly spin-
ning in an endless chain of thoughts, also needs rest. In our times,
the concept of rejuvenation and maintenance of the body is almost
nonexistent.

People maintain their houses; they have them painted and
repaired every now and then. They maintain their vehicles with
regular servicing. Yet if people are unable to sleep, they rarely
make an effort to bring order again to their lost rhythm, instead
relying on sleeping pills. The same can be said about many other
vital functions of the body and their related disorders. People today
seem to have a complete lack of knowledge about restoring the natural functions of the body.

Sexuality is no exception. Many people suffer from sexual problems simply because their general body equilibrium has been lost.

It is important that you learn that the first priority of life is life
itself. And therefore do not neglect yourself and spend too much
time on family responsibilities. Be conscious of your duty, but do
not forget that ensuring your physical and mental well-being is
your primary and sacred duty.

३. कायाकल्प के लिए नियमित रूप से पंचकर्म क्रियाएं, योगाभ्यास,
    बलवर्धक, द्रव्यों का उपयोग इत्यादि करना चाहिए।

**3. Regular cleansing practices, yogic practices, and intake of
    appropriate rejuvenating products are the principal meth-
    ods of rejuvenation.**

The subject of rejuvenation could be the theme of an entire
book. Although the process of human degeneration is irreversible,
it is up to us to lessen it or increase it. The first thing you can do
to rejuvenate yourself is to adopt the cleansing practices described
earlier in Part VI.[4] These practices help keep the body humors in

equilibrium, flush out toxins, purify blood, and increase ojas. In other words, they remove the hindrances in the way of sexuality and enhance physical attraction, making the skin smooth and shiny, giving luster to the body, and removing any unpleasant smell.

All these cleansing practices help diminish the process of degeneration by cleaning the energy channels and increasing the flow of energy in the body. Sexual problems or other illnesses are the results of negligence over a long period of time. People do not take their minor disorders seriously, and they go on "curing" them only symptomatically. Finally, one day the body becomes sluggish in its vital functions, and a major disease appears. Let me give you an example. Imagine a woman who has infrequent or partial evacuation. She does not think that it is an ailment and does not do anything about it. Not attending to this over a period of time, the vata in her body vitiates. This problem slowly increases and also becomes the cause of suffering during her pregnancy. It may also give rise to hemorrhoids, especially after delivery. During youth, she may still be able to tolerate the effects of vata vitiation, but with age, she will gradually begin to suffer from vata-related ailments, such as drying of sexual excretions, lack of power of retention, insomnia or other sleep disorders, pain in the body, fatigue, pain in the joints, arthritis, and so on. With all these health problems, enthusiasm and vigor for sexuality slowly diminish.

Had such a woman regularly followed the cleansing practices and taken care with her diet, her vata condition would not have worsened. A regular enema done with vata-decreasing substances at the end of each season can control this problem at the earliest stage. Sexual problems cannot be separated from other health problems; the seat of all these is the body.

Besides following the cleansing practices, you can revitalize your body with the yogic practices detailed in Part VI. Rejuvenating products can also contribute—by supplying vital dietary elements, improving digestion, and absorption of nutrients.

REJUVENATION

During recent years, some of the individual Ayurvedic plants related to rejuvenation have become known outside of India. Plants recently advertised in the Western media are *Chibulic myrobalan* (harada in Hindi), *Emblica officinalis* (amala), *Tinospora cordifolia* (giloye), *Commiphora mukul* (guggul), *Terminalia bellirica* (baheda), and *Withania somnifera* (asvagandha). In modern science laboratories one hears about the "wonderful" properties of these substances—how they prevent aging and related ailments. This reductionist way of looking at the Ayurvedic practice and the obliviousness to other methods of rejuvenation besides these drugs are typical of modern medicine.

I wish to emphasize that the intake of rejuvenating products must not substitute for other methods of rejuvenation. Furthermore, there are many other rejuvenating products besides the few plants just mentioned. Also, single plants (or minerals or any other natural substances) are not very common or very effective for rejuvenation. Rejuvenation products generally contain many substances and are prepared according to specific instructions so that their vital elements are not lost. It should be understood that if you lead an unhealthy life while taking rejuvenating products, they will not be of much use. For example, Ayurvedic practice recommends that during meals you fill only two-thirds of your stomach with solids and liquids. Filling yourself more vitiates the humors—irrespective of the foods' caloric values. Taking rejuvenating products while stuffing yourself in this way is like adding fuel to a fire with one hand while dousing it with water with the other. In brief, it is essential to cultivate a healthy Ayurvedic lifestyle along with the intake of rejuvenating products.

Rejuvenation is a vast subject and constitutes one of the eight parts of Ayurveda.[5] There are many rejuvenating substances in nature, and they may vary according to geographical conditions. In the following list I describe some simple recipes, while trying to recognize the availability of products in different parts of the world.

1. Take 8 ounces (200 grams) of almonds with skin, and soak them in water for four to five hours or overnight. Remove the skin and let them dry. Place them in a jar, add 1 pound (400 grams) of honey, and mix these well. Leave the mixture for ten days, then add, in powdered form, 2 ounces (50 grams) of black pepper and 3 ounces (75 grams) each of asparagus, licorice, basil, and anise seed. Puree the mixture in a blender. Take 3 teaspoons every morning before breakfast.

2. Take 4 ounces (100 grams) each of almonds, cashew nuts, and rock candy crystals, plus 2 ounces (50 grams) anise and twenty black peppercorns. Powder or grind each ingredient separately and then mix them well and store the mixture in a closed jar. Take 1 tablespoonful of this every day with hot milk. If you do not drink hot milk, take it with hot water or tea.

3. Mix together 10 ounces (250 grams) each of carrots, apples, and amala, a fruit from the Himalayas with multiple medicinal qualities (if available), and cut them into small pieces. Add 1/2 cup (100 ml) water and 5 ounces (150 grams) sugar to the mixture and cook the mixture, covered, for about an hour, stirring it from time to time. Add water if necessary to prevent burning and sticking. Add to this cooked mixture the following ingredients, in powdered form: 3/4 ounce (20 grams) of cardamom, 3/8 ounce (10 grams) of vanshalocan (the raisin from bamboo), 3/8 ounce (10 grams) of mastic (the raisin of a tree called *Pistacia lentiscus*, which comes from southern Europe), 4 ounces (100 grams) of peeled almonds, and 2 ounces (50 grams) of harada (*Chibulic myrobalan*). Puree all these ingredients together and preserve the mixture in a silver container, or, if this is not possible, keep a piece of pure silver in the container and keep stirring it from time to time (do not use a piece of jewelry, since jewelry almost always contains alloys). In Ayurvedic medicine, we mix very thin silver foil into this puree. Take 3 to 4 teaspoons of this every day.

This preparation may be difficult to make outside the Indian continent, given the nonavailability of some of the ingredients mentioned. However, more and more Ayurvedic products are now being exported, and perhaps some of these items will soon become more widely available.

4. Put 2 pounds (1 kilogram) each of carrots and apples, cut into small pieces, into a pot with 1 cup (200 ml) of water, and cook them, covered and on a low flame, for fifteen minutes. Add about 1 pound (1/2 kilo) of sugar and continue to cook the mixture for about an hour, stirring from time to time, until it becomes a thick paste. Let it cool, then add the following ingredients in powdered form: 1 ounce (25 grams) each of cardamom, clove, cinnamon, basil, dried ginger, laurel or bay leaves, ajwain or thyme seeds, and dill seeds. Also add fifty black peppercorns, almost 2 ounces (40 grams) each of cumin and anise; and 3 ounces (70 grams) of amala, harada (*Chibulic myrobalan*), and baheda. After mixing all the ingredients thoroughly, add just over 1 pound (500 grams) of honey, which acts as a preservative. Take 2 teaspoonfuls every morning or before going to bed.

You may make this preparation without amala, harada, and baheda if these are not available; but in this case, take a double dose. An equal mixture of the dried fruits of amala, harada, and baheda is called triphala (literally meaning "three fruits"). It helps to establish the equilibrium of the humors and is a very effective general tonic. A teaspoon of it can also be taken as such every day with honey or left to stand in a glass of water overnight and drunk the following morning. These days, many Ayurvedic products are available in the West, and it is quite possible that you may find triphala marketed as such in health-food stores.

5. Garlic is a rejuvenating product as well as an aphrodisiac. The daily dose of garlic is 1 to 4 grams, or two to three medium cloves, but you should be cautious: start with a small clove and then increase the dose up to three cloves. Garlic can be hard to digest, so take it only according to your constitution and digestive power. Stop taking it if it gives you digestive problems, excessive thirst, and restlessness. Find out your constitution according to the charts given in Part III and take garlic as follows. If you are a vata person, take crushed garlic with a teaspoon of ghee. Do not drink anything cold for at least an hour after taking it. If you are a pitta person, crush garlic in a teaspoon of rock candy crystals and drink a glass of cold water afterwards. Kapha persons should crush the garlic and mix it with a teaspoon of honey.

The best way to fight the strong smell of garlic is to chew five to six cardomoms daily. Cardamom has many other positive effects on health. (For details, see my book *Ayurveda: A Way of Life*.)

6. Saffron is also a rejuvenating product, as already mentioned. For the rejuvenating effect, mix 1 ounce (25 grams) with 2 ounces (50 grams) each of rock candy crystals and ghee and whip it thoroughly. Take 1/2 teaspoon of this every day with hot milk. If you do not drink milk, just eat the mixture as such, or try hot water or hot tea. Do not drink anything cold after it for at least an hour.

A Reminder About Ingredients

Nuts should be bought raw without being subjected to any treatment and almonds always with the skin on. Be careful when you buy other herbs and spices that they are not too old. Do not buy them in powdered form. They lose their value with time and much more quickly once ground or powdered. You can easily grind them yourself with a small coffee grinder kept exclusively for this purpose, unless a hand grinder is specified. Before grinding, make sure that the herbs and spices are clean (remove any stones, etc.). Put them briefly in the sun or in a low-heated oven before grinding. For more details on the pharmaceutical properties of many of these ingredients, methods of making fine powders, decoctions, or other details concerning general preparations, you may consult my book Ayurveda: A Way of Life.

४. कायाकल्प मानसिक स्तर पर भी आवश्यक है।

4. Rejuvenation of the mind is equally essential.

Each person should have a few minutes of silence and concentration immediately after getting up in the morning and before sleeping at night, accompanied by pranayama practices. You can also rejuvenate the mind by abiding with the simple code of conduct—to stay concentrated on the one thing that you are doing at any given moment of time.

Sleep rejuvenates both body and mind, so ensure yourself appropriate sleep. Too much sleep is as bad as too little. Adults should not sleep more than seven to eight hours each night, and they should avoid day sleep except during summer afternoons. Too much sleep leads to lethargy and indifference to sexual desire.

The mind can also be rejuvenated with a head massage using special oils meant for this purpose, such as amala or Brahmi or Bhringraja oils. If such oils are not available, you can substitute almond or sesame oil. Different types of nuts, especially cashews and almonds, help revitalize the brain and should be included in your diet during the winter months. White pumpkin seeds are nerve strengthening.

५. इन सब उपचारों से सुख और पूर्णता का अनुभव होता है।

5. Rejuvenation creates a feeling of well-being and fulfillment.

A regularly rejuvenated body and mind yield a sense of well-being, a pleasant disposition, and an attractive appearance. This gives rise to a liberal and free attitude towards life, harmonious relationships with one's surroundings, and an appropriate sense of time and space. With these come intuition and wisdom.

६. काम में शारीरिक परिपूर्णता तथा गहन अनुभव के लिए यह उपचार आवश्यक हैं।

6. These methods of rejuvenation are fundamental for sensual fulfillment and experiencing the depth of sexual union.

For complete sensuous fulfillment and a profound experience of sexuality, both partners must express themselves spontaneously, without restrictions and restraint, and this is only possible if they both share a sense of well-being within themselves and are in harmony with their environments.

७. बाजीकरण का ठीक अर्थ तथा महत्त्व समझ लेना चाहिए।

7. Aphrodisiacs must be understood correctly and used appropriately.

The word *aphrodisiac* is generally misunderstood today, and aphrodisiacs themselves are often misused. Many people think that aphrodisiacs are mysterious substances that wildly increase one's sexual potential. And some people make a big business out of selling so-called aphrodisiacs without any specificity to cure sexual problems. True aphrodisiacs, however, vary greatly and are supposed to function at different levels and aspects of sexuality. Though they range widely, all aphrodisiacs enhance one or more of the following: sexual impulse, duration of the sexual act, sexual vigor, sexual excretion, or sexual attraction. They may be divided into four major categories: (1) aphrodisiacs that increase sexual secretions, enhance the quality of semen, and promote fertility; (2) aphrodisiacs that enhance sexual excitement and vigor; (3) aphrodisiacs that help prolong sexual activity; and (4) aphrodisiacs that increase both sexual excretions and excitement.

Substances, actions, or factors which diminish sexual vigor, fertility, and so on may be termed *anaphrodisiacs* (I coined this word by translating from Sanskrit). Removal of anaphrodisiacs is essential before application of any aphrodisiac. In fact, many problems in sexuality can be attributed to the hindrances caused by factors and situations which act as anaphrodisiacs.

In ancient texts, aphrodisiacs and their effects are mostly described for men, and when women are mentioned, the focus is all on fertility and lactation. It is not that ancient Indians thought that women did not enjoy sexuality or did not have orgasms; they simply took a one-sided view on such topics. Perhaps they thought a man's ability, cleverness, and vigor were all that was needed to evoke a woman's sexual expression.

Several ancient treatises on sex also state that women have eight times more sexual energy than men and that an attractive woman is the most effective aphrodisiac. I have also discussed this subject with some Ayurvedic physicians or *vaidyas* who think that, besides appropriate care after giving birth, women do not need any aphrodisiacs. It may well be that ancient male writers thought that woman, the source of sexual energy, could not possibly need something to enhance it.

I feel that this view not only ignores women but also fails to consider men who have a larger percentage of female principle, who may be unable to lead a woman in a sexual relationship. A woman too should be taught ways to modify her sexual expression according to the qualities of her partner.

Perhaps the question of women and aphrodisiacs was too complicated for the ancient sages, or perhaps the ethnic tradition that leaves most aspects of the care of women in the hands of women was too strong. This traditional wisdom was passed on orally from generation to generation, so there would have been no need for the sages to add to it.

ट. देश, काल और आवश्यकता के अनुसार ही बाजीकरण पदार्थों का सेवन करना चाहिए।

8. Use of aphrodisiacs should be appropriate to time, place, and need.

A person with normal health and energy does not usually need to take aphrodisiacs. Removal of anaphrodisiacs and rejuvenating therapy help increase sexual vigor and retention. However, specific aphrodisiacs may help in certain circumstances and life situations. The "time" referred to in the sutra means both one's age and the time of the year. For example, during youth, sexual desire and secretions are in abundance, and aphrodisiacs should not be taken without any specific need. Besides, in each case, one should first try to remove the hindrances in sexual expression before beginning to use aphrodisiacs.

There are times in a woman's life when she requires aphrodisiacs, specifically, after childbirth or during the premenopausal period. The state of shock common at these times may have negative effects on both men and women. An aphrodisiac therapy and counseling from a good holistic physician can help in such cases.

A couple should pay attention to their sexual behavior and the changes taking place with time. They should make an effort to renew and refresh their relationship. If they feel they are having less and less of a sexual relationship, they should immediately attend to this situation by talking about it and taking measures to improve it. Delay always makes a situation worse and may make it more complicated.

When people stay together a long time, it seems that their sexuality often withers away, perhaps from boredom and neglect. This is where aphrodisiacs, coupled with some personal effort, can be important. In such a situation as a traditional family, a woman generally suffers more, since men most often begin to have relationships outside. A woman with children generally feels more committed and she cannot afford to have another relationship. Remember that aphrodisiacs are not only products but also all other factors that enhance sexuality—for example, massage, body care, dressing up, smelling good, and so on. Pay attention to the rhythm and variety in your sexuality, and take appropriate aphrodisiac measures to maintain the sexual relationship with your partner.

Aphrodisiac substances should be suitable to the circumstances and climatic conditions of a given place and should not give rise to side effects. For example, garlic is an aphrodisiac which increases sexual secretions and vigor. But do not take it in a hot climate, and take it only in an appropriate way, so that it does not create side effects like excessive thirst or restlessness. Asparagus is also an aphrodisiac, but it is cold in nature and so should not be taken too much in the winter. In fact, the balanced preparation of asparagus described here would not produce side effects.

Aphrodisiacs should be used according to need and circumstance. Some people are weak in their sexual expression and vigor and are unable to have a prolonged union. Others may have a psychological blockage due to religious beliefs or some other external influence. Some women may need something to help them reach the peak of sexual expression, whereas some men may need measures for prolonging sexual activity. Some good aphrodisiac preparations act on sexual excretions, endurance, and vigor simultaneously. Women may lack vaginal secretion and men an erection. Aphrodisiac measures can be useful in all such cases, after a proper rejuvenating therapy.

METHODS FOR THE PREPARATION OF SOME APHRODISIAC PRODUCTS

1. Almonds have an aphrodisiac effect, but a specific preparation is required. After soaking the almonds overnight in water and peeling off the skin, pound the almonds for a very long time, until they turn into a paste so fine that if you smear a little bit of it on your skin, it will be partly absorbed. Prepare this paste with a stone pestle and mortar and not with an electric grinder of any sort. Add to it an equal quantity of honey and mix well. Take 3 to 4 teaspoons of this preparation with hot milk every day. Hot cow's milk and ghee also have an aphrodisiac effect.

Since this preparation holds its value over time, you can make larger quantities: for example, with 8 ounces (200 grams) each of almonds and honey. But to reach the kind of fine paste you want, you'll have to take small quantities of almonds at one time.

2. Take 4 ounces (100 grams) of fresh, good-quality garlic. After removing the skin, pound it and add in 8 ounces (200 grams) of honey. Put this preparation in a closed jar and put it away to ripen in a cupboard, away from any heat source, for twenty-one days. Take 1/2 teaspoon daily. (Since garlic is light, it floats on the surface, and you'll have to stir the mixture for half a minute every day with a spoon before closing the jar again. Lessen the quantity if you have side effects. See the box accompanying Sutra 3 for more about garlic, its side effects, and ways to get rid of its odor.

3. Fine powder of licorice should be taken with ghee and honey. For a single dose, take 1 teaspoon of this powder, add 1 teaspoon each of ghee and honey, and mix all the ingredients.

4. Soak 4 ounces (100 grams) of amala powder in 2/3 cup (150 ml) of water overnight. Strain this liquid through a muslin cloth (you may throw away the solids or use them as compost). Add another 4 ounces (100 grams) of fine amala powder to this concentrate and mix it well. Spread the mixture in a plate or tray, and dry it in the sun. Mix this preparation with 2 tablespoons each of ghee, rock candy crystals, and honey. Take 2 teaspoons every day.

5. Urad beans (like mung beans in shape, but black instead of green) have tremendous aphrodisiac qualities. While mung beans can act as a cure for vitiated humors, urad beans are a strong food and can create humor imbalance unless prepared in specific combinations. Following is an example:

Take 8 ounces (200 grams) of beans without the skins (they

are easily available in Indian foodshops all over the world). Clean them and check for stones and so on, and then wash them well six to seven times with water. (If you can get only beans with the skin on, soak them for three to four hours in water, then take off the skin.)

Drain all the water from the washed beans and soak them in 2/3 cup (150 ml) of milk previously sweetened with 2 ounces (50 grams) of sugar. Leave this for five to six hours or overnight. In a hot climate without air conditioning, reduce this time to two or three hours.

Mash this in a blender or grind it by hand and it will give rise to a thick and sticky batter. This batter can then be used to make something like thick pancakes or small, deep-fried balls. In either case, fry them in ghee.

The quantity just described is a three-day supply. Store the batter in the refrigerator and fry the pancakes or balls just before eating them. Since this is a rich dish, eat it instead of a meal.

This mixture can be made in large quantities and preserved. If you want to do that, make small flattened shapes with the batter, resembling cookies. Put them in plates smeared with butter or ghee, and place them in the sun until they are thoroughly dry. The drying period depends on the intensity of the sun. (Or try using the oven in colder climates.) In a dried form, they can be preserved for several months at room temperature. Deep fry them in ghee shortly before eating.

6. Two teaspoons of dried, powdered asparagus should be taken with hot sweetened milk every day. Sweeten the milk with sugar, not honey, which should never be heated, according to Ayurvedic wisdom. During the asparagus-growing season, cut the stalks into small pieces and dry them for a long-lasting supply. Do not try to substitute asparagus root for the dried stalks.

7. Nutmeg is suggested for those who are nervous and hectic in nature. Men should take it to prolong their sexual capacity. A daily dose is 1/2 gram of a ground or grated fruit (about one-fourth of a medium-sized nutmeg). You can eat nutmeg in a soup or with other prepared food or else gulp it down with a glass of warm water.

Nutmeg paste is also used to cure impotence. First reduce it to a fine powder in a mortar and pestle or stone grinder, then add sesame oil until you have a very fine paste. The paste can be smeared directly on the penis every day and left several hours or overnight. In fact, the paste dries up fast and falls off by itself.

Another way to cure impotence is to wrap a beetle leaf smeared with nutmeg crude oil around the penis, with the help of a bandage, and to leave this overnight.

8. Some women have problems reaching the peak of their sexual expression and may wish to decrease this time period to be more compatible with their male partners. A mixture of jaggery, tamarind fruit pulp, and a small quantity of pepper, smeared in the vagina can help you reach the peak of sexual expression rapidly, as well as increase sexual secretion. Mix 1 teaspoon each of crushed jaggery and tamarind pulp with one or two ground peppercorns.

9. To prolong sexual capacity and enhance sexual vigor, do not eat sour or excessively salty foods. Take foods with ghee and milk.

10. Use of sesame, coconut, and ginger in food increases sexual secretions.

Homeopathic remedies:

Please note that the "X" accompanying a numeral following the name of the medicine indicates the strength of the dilution of the substance; when you buy the homeopathic remedy, the pharmacist needs to have this indication of strength. In each instance, the "dose" consists of 3–4 pills or pellets.

a. *Agnus castus* should be taken when there are symptoms like abhorrence of sexual intercourse, yellow leukorrhea, and sexual melancholy. For males, it is given when there is no erection or no sexual desire. Dose: *Agnus castus* 6X, three times a day.

b. *Phosphoricum acidum* should be taken by a woman when she has no sexual desire after having given birth and when there is weakness due to breast-feeding.

c. *Natrum muriaticum* is given to cure diminished sexual desire due to some psychological reasons like fear, anxiety, suffering, or shock. Dose: *Natrum muriaticum* 200X, once every three days.

d. *Sepia* is given when there is a lack of sexual desire due to some pain in the vagina during intercourse. Dose: *Sepia* 200X, every other day.

---

६. बाजीकरण तथा कामसादक पदार्थ काम जीवन में सन्तुलन लाने के लिए प्रयोग किये जाने चाहिए।

9. Aphrodisiacs and anaphrodisiacs should be used to have a harmonious sexual companionship.

Sexual incompatibility between two partners can be very troublesome and may give rise to other problems. Incompatibility may also develop due to variations in sexual behavior, as when one has tremendous sexual vigor and the other has less. Such cases may be handled with the use of aphrodisiacs or anaphrodisiacs. These latter are especially necessary for those with excessive sexual vigor.

The noble aim of taking aphrodisiac measures should be to develop communication at the physical, mental, and spiritual levels during sexual union. If you use aphrodisiacs merely to display your sexual capability, you will only create an imbalance by diverting most of your vitality in this direction, and you will weaken yourself.

Some people who have excessive sexual desire think that by taking something to cure it, they will become incapacitated for sex-

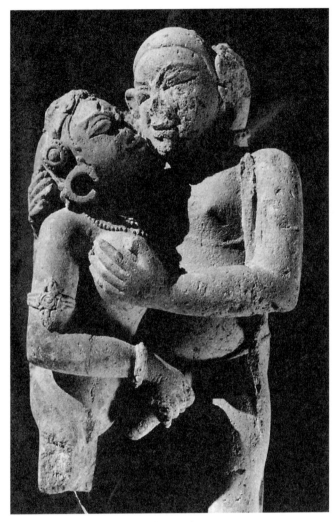

Erotic couple.

ual performance. They should realize that this excess denotes a disequilibrium in their bodies, which over a long period of time may lead to a serious disease. People who have this problem are generally suffering from pitta vitiation and may also have digestive disorders. It is essential to cure such a disorder without delay. An appropriate internal cleansing and the use of rejuvenating products may bring back the lost balance. Excessive sexual energy can also be channeled through yogic methods, as described in Part IX, Sutra 3.

══════ ANAPHRODISIAC PRODUCTS ══════

The simplest and most easily available anaphrodisiac product is coriander. Seeds should be taken in powdered form. Take a teaspoonful daily for a few days and repeat if necessary. Take care that the coriander seeds you buy are not too old. If you are not able to take the powdered seed straight, make a tea by mixing 1 teaspoonful in 1 cup (250 ml) of water and boiling over a low heat until reduced by half. Filter and drink.

Herbal drugs with a bitter taste generally have an anaphrodisiac effect. People with excessive sexual desire should avoid eating too much ginger, garlic, other spices with pungent tastes, meat soup, and old sweet wine, among other foods.

———

९०. कायाकल्प में प्रयुक्त होने वाले पदार्थ ओजस को बढ़ाने के कारण बाजीकरण भी हो सकते हैं।

10. Rejuvenating products may also have an aphrodisiac effect.

Many people have the mistaken notion that rejuvenating products are aphrodisiacs. Rejuvenation, however, is an important part of Ayurveda and an entire therapy: it is not limited only to products.

Nevertheless, in individual cases, the various measures of rejuvenation therapy may act as aphrodisiacs. Such therapy may bring back into balance the body's humors, improving sexual performance. Further, rejuvenating products increase ojas in the body. With this increase of general energy level, sexual performance becomes more vigorous, and capacity to prolong the sexual union may increase. When general vitality is low, people usually gather all their energy to put into their work; one is not left with much choice. Besides the means of livelihood, for many people work is also connected to fame, name, and prestige. After work, they are exhausted and need rest to regain their energy for the next day's work. What usually suffers most is sexuality. Rejuvenating products enhance the body's vitality not only because they contain elements vital to life but also because they regulate digestion and enhance assimilation of nutrients.

Massage is both rejuvenating and an aphrodisiac. In our hectic times, vata tends to dominate, due to excessive activity and wrong nutrition. Massage brings this humor into equilibrium, strengthens the nerves, and opens energy channels. In the present context, massage should not be understood as something for a temporary sexual excitement. On the contrary, it should help one to come to a restful mental state so that one can participate in sexual activities with great vigor and enthusiasm. Its purpose is not to turn the sexual energy into a spark which comes with a great speed and dies out very fast but rather to enhance the sexual expression and retention. It should be done with the aim to bring the other person to a state of complete relaxation.

If sexual expression is hindered due to general fatigue, a whole-body massage will be very helpful. Otherwise, the important points of massage for the present purpose are palms, soles, ears, toes, both sides of the lower part of the neck region, and the spinal region. This latter is especially important because of the location of the concentric energy points. Massage the whole vertebral column by pressing and making round movements at each vertebra. Later, concentrate the massage in a similar way on the sites of the five chakras which are located along the spine (see Fig. 28).

११. बाजीकरण पदार्थों के प्रयोग से पहले जो कुछ कामसादक हो उसको दूर करना चाहिए।

11. Before using any aphrodisiac, remove all anaphrodisiacs.

If you don't remove all factors that will become a hindrance to sexual expression before you use aphrodisiacs, the aphrodisiacs will be hardly or not at all effective. This would be like putting oil on the fire with one hand and water on with the other.

Diverse factors may act as anaphrodisiacs. Sexual attitude, overwork, fatigue, exhaustion, restless mind, thoughts about another person, lack of appropriate atmosphere, fear, use of sedatives or some other drugs, a hectic mechanized lifestyle, lack of respect and appreciation for one's partner, general weakness of the body, lack of ojas, negative previous experiences or a negative exposure to sexuality, the reading and watching of pornographic material, and sexual fantasies are some noted anaphrodisiac factors.

To get rid of all that hinders the flow of sexual energy, first find out the exact problem. If you develop your strength of mind with the methods already described, you will be able to diagnose your problems yourself, which is better than seeking any outside counseling. Most people are unable to do this because, instead of looking for the real problem and its solution, they spend most of their time blaming others for what has happened to them. This increases the problem instead of solving it. Modern psychology has done great harm to the Western mind in this respect.

Before using aphrodisiacs, you should undergo an inner cleansing. In Ayurveda, it is stated that just like a dirty cloth does not absorb a dye properly, so aphrodisiac products are a waste if taken without proper evacuation.[6]

═══════ PERFUMING THE VAGINA ═══════

It is unpleasant to have a bad smell from the vagina, just as it is from the mouth. Besides the effect on sexual interaction, it is unhealthy and disagreeable for you to have an offensive smell. Therefore, if this happens, it should be immediately attended to. The bad odor may be due to some foods because in women, this is another area, like the armpits, for the release of certain substances consumed by the body. Here are some simple measures for getting rid of vaginal odor.

1. Heat 2 teaspoons of ghee and mix into it one ground clove and two ground cardamoms. Let it cook for half a minute on low heat. When it cools down to an appropriate temperature, you can apply the oil to the vaginal walls and the vaginal opening to create a pleasant smell.

2. Diluted sandalwood oil or a paste made from its wood by rubbing it on a stone, or diluted anise oil may be used to smear the vaginal area to get a pleasant smell. If you want to use an essential oil, simply dilute a drop of oil with 1 ounce (2 tablespoons) of water.

3. Some perfumed flowers like jasmine, rose, and lavender can be cooked on low heat in sesame oil to obtain perfumed oil. Use 2 ounces (50 grams) of flowers per 1/2 cup of heated sesame oil, cooked on a low flame for ten minutes. Or you can simply dilute an essential oil—one part oil to ten parts sesame oil.

The resulting perfumed oil should be applied to the vaginal walls and vulva.

───────────────────────────────

नारी कामसूत्र के दसवें भाग की यहां इति होती है। इसमें कायाकल्प और बाजीकरण विधियों पर प्रकाश डाला गया है।

This brings to an end Part X of *The Kamasutra for Women*, about rejuvenation and aphrodisiacs.

PART XI
*S*exuality and *S*piriituality

. . .

ग्यारहवाँ भाग

काम का आत्मज्ञान से सम्बन्ध

. . .

A sage partakes the sensuous pleasures as they occur with
a detached mind and does not become addicted to desire.

—*Gopala-Uttara-Tapini Upanishad*

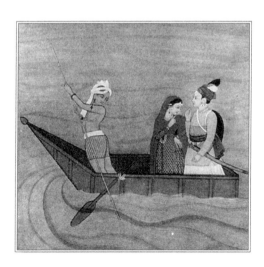

९. काम में इन्द्रियाँ बहुत गहन रूप से अपने विषयों में आसक्त होती हैं।

1. Sexuality is the most intense of all the sensuous experiences.

Sexuality is the most intense sensuous experience because all five senses are simultaneously involved to their maximum capacity during the sexual act. One may say that there is a spontaneous flow of sexual energy during sexual expression. However, if there are hindrances to sexual expression, the intensity decreases. For example, rough skin, an offensive smell, or an unpleasant taste can become an obstacle to passionate kissing. A mosquito bite can cause a sudden interruption. So try to remove the possible obstacles at the onset of sexual activity.

A unique feature of sexuality is the involvement of two persons, each with an expression of his or her five senses: an orchestra of five pairs of senses intercommunicating simultaneously at individual and joint levels.

During sexual activity, the senses reach a peak of expression, then come to a state where all action ceases. The sexual experience consists of three stages, corresponding to the three fundamental qualities of the Cosmic Substance—rajas, tamas, and sattva (Fig. 35). Sexual preparation and activity, including beautifying oneself to be sexually attractive, and most parts of the sexual act itself indicate rajas. After this intense sexual activity comes a phase of tamas when the activity begins to cease because the senses cannot go on any more. After this brief state of tamas, one enters into the last phase of sexuality—a moment of beatitude, an experience of pure consciousness. During this state, the mind dwells in its sattva element and becomes one with the soul instead of identifying itself with the senses. This moment has been described in ancient texts as *Brahmananda*, the joy of experiencing the Supreme Soul or the Absolute. At this point, one has transcended the senses and

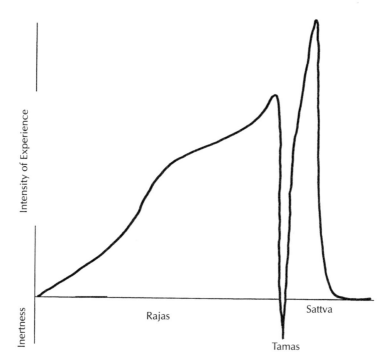

Figure 35   The phases of sexual experience vary in terms of the three fundamental qualities.

reached that immense state of pure energy which is the cause of our being.

To transcend the senses, one must first experience them intensely. This is true not only for sexuality but also in yoga. For example, an excessively intense experience of one particular sense leads to a state too intense to tolerate, so that one transcends that very state and achieves a thought-free mind. Like this, the activities of the mind are silenced and an experience of stillness is achieved.

An adept of yoga makes a long-term effort to achieve a state when she or he is able to transcend the senses through the efforts of the mind. Similarly, the period of rajas in sexuality is very long.

Activity reaches a peak, and there is a brief but intense sense of exhaustion—the phase of tamas. After this, one enters into the state of sattva.

२. इस आसक्ति के बाद किंचित आनन्द की अनुभूति होती है जिसमें आत्मभाव का अनुभव होता है।

2. Sexuality leads to a momentary beatitude—a brief experience of pure consciousness.

When all the action of the senses ceases, there remains nothing. One reaches a state of void which is immense and indescribable and is accompanied by an intense bliss. One cannot say that it is a "feeling" of bliss, as at that particular moment there is no feeling. One experiences the beatitude, and its realization comes after that particular moment.

The mind has a continuous chain of thoughts all the time. Although it is closed to new knowledge during sleep as the senses are at rest, the thought process keeps flowing in the form of dreams, or in nothing more than the realization of sleep being good or bad. One can stop the chain of thoughts through various yogic practices. The same state is achieved temporarily with sexual experience.

According to the philosophy of yoga, the mind is both the cause of involvement in the world and the pathway for withdrawal from the world to the state of pure consciousness. However, the aim of yoga is not to have a brief experience of pure consciousness, but its ultimate realization. Through sexuality, we momentarily achieve oneness with the cause of being. Technically, it is similar to the yogic experience, but it is very brief.

३. मानसिक प्रयत्न द्वारा इन्द्रियों के चरम अनुभव से अतीत होकर मनुष्य को आत्मज्ञान का अनुभव होता है।

3. A spiritual experience is one that is beyond sensuous experience and can be achieved by transcending the senses with the efforts of the mind.

The cause of being is the soul, which is itself only energy. It is not involved in the world. It is like a reflecting glass or an onlooker who does not participate in any activity but views the scene without being involved. Normally, we identify ourselves with our physical being because it has form, shape, color, and so on. However, the real self of an individual is the soul that breathes life into the body of the five senses.

When the mind withdraws from the senses through its own efforts and comes to a state of stillness, it acquires the nature of the soul, which is still, inactive, and uninvolved. This experience is termed a spiritual experience. Spiritual experience is achieved only by transcending the senses.

४. प्रयत्न तथा अभ्यास से आत्मानुभूति द्वारा प्राप्त आनन्द का अनुभव बढ़ाया जा सकता है।

4. Through personal effort and practice, the experience of beatitude can be prolonged.

Sexuality leads to a momentary beatitude, an experience of pure consciousness, a state in which the mind is still and identifies itself with the cause of being—the soul. What one achieves through sexuality is a very short-lived experience of spirituality. The senses express themselves completely, and then their activity ceases, there is a stillness and an experience of void, and the mind becomes one with the soul—the cause of consciousness. Our physical, mutable self dissolves for a moment into our real, immortal self.

This state of beatitude can be prolonged through personal effort and constant practice. Normally, the short-lived state of beatitude is a natural outcome of sexuality. Everybody likes it, enjoys it, and finds it exhilarating. Technically, even the short-lived experience is spiritual, but it is too brief to have such a certain character. Our aim in talking about sexuality and spirituality is to prolong this experience through the efforts of the mind, through yogic methods of mind control. Everything begins at the point where stillness of the mind is already achieved.

५. बाह्य रूप तथा विचार आदि की भिन्नता होने पर भी हमारे अन्दर का जीव या आत्मा, जो जीवन शक्ति का कारण है, सब में एक ही है तथा अपरिवर्तनीय और अविनाशी है।

5. **Despite differences in outward appearance, opinions, views, and so on, the indestructible and immutable energy which is the cause of consciousness is alike in all human beings.**

Some of you might think that the experience of spirituality through sexuality is the domain of only some few special people who are endowed with mental strength or have a high intellect or the like. Despite differences in our physical manifestations, the inner self is the same in all human beings. Whether we are black, white, or brown, rich or poor, whatever the means of our livelihood, whatever our educational qualifications, our honor, fame, or title, our bodies and minds are made of the same cosmic elements, and the energy which kindles life in us is the same. The variations in the organization of the five elements and the stock of our previous karma makes us different from one another in innumerable ways and manners. However, the light that keeps us alive is untouched by karma and its results. Its power does not diminish or increase in any circumstances. The sufferings or pleasures resulting from karma are worn by the physical self. To have a spiritual experience, we have to transcend the physical self bound to time and to the results of constant change in the phenomenal universe due to karma, and to be one with the cause of being. Since this latter is the same in all of us, the path to spirituality is equally open for all human beings. This does not mean that some may not need more effort and mental training than others to achieve this goal.

६. काम द्वारा आत्मज्ञान का अनुभव करने के लिए इन्द्रियों की पूरी आसक्ति आवश्यक है।

6. Reaching a spiritual experience through sexuality requires a complete immersion into sensuality.

Complete immersion in the sensuous experience is necessary if you ultimately intend to transcend the senses. Your attention should not be diverted during sexual congress. All effort of both the mind and the body should be concentrated on the details of your physical self and the subtle feelings of the other person. During sexual congress, nothing else should be important: that span of time is the most precious moment of your life. You are there and only there. Forget that a world exists outside your little environment.

To practice this concentration will require considerable time and effort. You might question why we need this complete sensual immersion if what we're aiming at is spirituality. It is through sensuality that we have to reach the cosmic energy within ourselves. Sensuality is merely a path, not the aim. If it is not intense, pleasant, enjoyable, and fulfilling, we may get entangled in this state only and never be able to reach the aim.

The heightened state of sensuous experience that arrives when you are fully immersed also helps you achieve full concentration of the mind. The more the mind is still, the more you're able to plunge into sensuous intensity. Mental strength and sensuous intensity enhance and strengthen each other.

Another factor important for an intense and smooth sensuous expression is the power to prolong sexual congress. In a short sexual session, it is not possible to have a complete expression of the senses. The intensity increases slowly during sexual communication, and the enhanced state of intensity should last for some time until the sensuous expression is exhausted and action ceases. A sexual congress which does not last long creates a kind of tension and insecurity in the two persons involved, an insecurity which further diminishes the intensity of expression. In other words, if you cannot have full expression and pleasure at the physical level, you cannot aspire to a deep experience of spirituality.

७. काम द्वारा आत्मज्ञान प्राप्त करने के लिए चित्त की एकाग्रता, शरीर का लचीलापन तथा प्राणायाम का अभ्यास आवश्यक हैं।

7. **Concentration of mind, flexibility of body, and mastery of breathing practices are needed to have a spiritual experience through sexuality.**

This sutra emphasizes that spirituality is not a theme to be taken independently of what has already been said about sexuality in this book.

Pranayama practices are essential for controlling the mind and should also be used to prolong the moment of beatitude. Just as the senses come to their peak of expression and are about to enter a state of inaction, concentrate fully on the state of beatitude you are about to enter. Direct your *pranashakti* ("power of life"—i.e., the air you inhale) towards your head at the moment you are going to enter into the domain of stillness. After doing this, try to prolong the spiritual experience by concentrating on the solar plexus, the site of the anahata chakra (see Part VII). This chakra, the fourth from the bottom, symbolizes the ultimate union and ful-fillment of male and female principles.

Each person will have a different experience in the beginning, due to variations in karma. However, with regular practice, the residues of previous karma will gradually dissolve, and you will attain spiritual lucidity. If you have reached this step successfully, you will be guided by the light of your individual soul to the realm of immensity, which is the Absolute and the Universal Soul.

A repeated, regular practice for developing singlepointedness of mind is needed to attain spiritual experience, which is possible only if you have obtained mastery over your mind and have a healthy and energetic body. The effort to experience spirituality through sexuality involves applying what you have already achieved with long-time practice. The main hindrance on the way to success is that, engrossed in the sensuous experience, you will tend not to discriminate among various stages of the sexual experience and will get lost in the means themselves. The state of rajas is very long, while tamas and sattva are more intense, but very brief.

८. इन्द्रियों से अतीत अनुभव करने का ध्येय मन में रखकर काम से इन्द्रियों की आसक्ति बढ़ानी चाहिए।

8. To achieve spiritual experience, proceed with the goal of transcending the senses.

Proceed with the aim of spiritual experience from the very beginning. Firm determination to experience the reality beyond the senses should guide your pursuit of sensuous intensity. Enhance the sensuous with this goal in mind. Enhancing sensuousness for the pure physical pleasure is something quite different, and doing this will not produce a spiritual experience as a by-product.

It already requires a long practice and a strong will for a couple to enhance sensuous intensity so that they can reach the point of harmony where all of their senses have oneness in their rhythm. It is essential to attain mastery at this level before aspiring to an experience of spirituality.

Progress in learning to transcend the physical is very slow. But with appropriate devotion and will, you will notice constant progress. You have to learn to transcend your own physical self as well as your partner's. If you have the slightest consciousness of the other person at the moment of beatitude, you are still in the phenomenal world. You have to traverse that and reach the state where all feelings cease. Next is the state of "no more feelings"—an experience of pure void.

CHANNELING SEXUAL ENERGY DURING SEXUAL COMMUNICATION

This process is more elaborate and requires a tremendous amount of training as compared to channeling sexual impulse. During sexual communication, the sexual energy is scattered in all parts of the body, and you have to continuously accumulate and direct it for a specific purpose. The sensuous pleasure is evoked with various activities through tactile sensation, the senses of smell and taste, loving language, admiration, and observation of the interplay of all these actions. These activities give rise to a tremendous amount of pleasure. However, this pleasure does not appear in a continuum but in periodic rhythm like the waves of the sea. Each time, the sense of joy has to be directed upwards to the mind or to the solar plexus. It requires a constant effort of the mind to prevent yourself from getting lost in this joy at a very mundane physical level. As compared to directing the sexual impulse, this method is difficult; in the former, a package of energy is transported, whereas in the latter, the scattered bits of energy are accumulated from various parts and transported each time. On the other hand, this process gives you a tremendous amount of pleasure at another level than physical. You have the sense of satisfaction the same way, but it is not like a release of energy accompanied by a feeling of exhaustion. On the contrary, it is enriching and gives a feeling of strength and force.

This method can be especially beneficial when you feel insecure about your partner and you have an unstable relationship. By using this yogic method, the other person becomes the least important element and you acquire a tremendous amount of strength. The other person is there for you but yet not there. His or her physical reality is a medium for your activities, but you stop feeling the indispensability of this particular being and, thus, insecurity vanishes. You acquire a mental state that an adept of yoga aims at. You retain a body and your senses and all the worldly actions are done through them. But your state of mind becomes transparent to the world's activities, which are perceived through the senses.

६. इन्द्रियों से परे का अनुभव आत्मदर्शन होता है।

9. The experience beyond senses leads to spiritual lucidity.

The experience beyond senses is the experience of immensity and oneness with the cosmic energy. This experience leads to the realization of one's true self—the soul and its unity with the cosmic power of being. This is a state of spiritual lucidity. A spiritual experience, whether obtained through sexuality or with yogic methods, leads us to perceive more than what we can with our senses. The domain of reality becomes wider, leading to a better comprehension of life and the cosmos, giving us discriminating knowledge to foresee events and to act wisely. The spiritual lucidity becomes a guiding force in our life, providing a blissful state of equilibrium and the strength and energy to rise above happy and unhappy life situations.

१०. आत्मदर्शन से अनन्तता का अनुभव होता है।

10. Spiritual lucidity leads to the experience of the infinite.

Repeated experience of spiritual lucidity leads us to identify with the real self, the soul. The soul is an immense source of energy, since it is a part of the universal energy. Thus, repeated spiritual experience connects us to the infinite cosmic energy.

११. आत्मज्ञान से प्राप्त असीमित शक्ति का प्रयोग मानव कल्याण के लिए करना चाहिए।

11. Spiritual energy may be directed for the well-being of humanity.

Spiritual energy thus obtained may be used in healing ailments, giving courage, and showing the right path to others. To use spiritual energy for a specific purpose, concentrate on the object concerned during the time of beatitude. For example, if you want to heal yourself, direct your prana to that part just as you are about to enter the moment of beatitude. If you want to achieve a bigger purpose, such as success in something, concentrate on that particular theme the same way. Just superficially thinking won't work—you must immerse the moment of beatitude with the purpose you want to achieve.

Spiritual energy can also be used for other purposes—to achieve material gains, to manipulate others for your own benefit, to take revenge, and so on. However, misuse of the spiritual energy leads to afflictions, the loss of peace of mind, and, eventually, to loss of the spiritual lucidity itself. On the other hand, using energy for the well-being of humanity brings courage, strength, and peace.

CHANNELING SEXUAL ENERGY
FOR A SPECIFIC PURPOSE

Whatever may be the purpose, the method applies to all cases. Let us take an example: You want to use your sexual energy for a creative purpose—it may be painting, designing, writing, or anything else. For this, do the same as just described, but this time you are pulling up your sexual impulse while concentrating on the essence of your work. This aim should be kept in mind before you actually begin the precise method.

Sexual energy can also be directed for preventing an ailment one is afraid of. It is used for making a protective armor (*kavacha*) around yourself. This means that you concentrate on the force of sexual impulse and direct it to encircle your body with the help of profound, or rapid, pranayama. Do this practice regularly, and whenever you are fearful, close your eyes and visualize the protective covering around you. Tell yourself repeatedly that this strong armor around you will expel any evil force which may cause disharmony and disturbance in your life. This method can also be used to develop courage and get over any kind of fear.

नारी कामसूत्र के अन्तिम भाग की इति होती है। इसमें काम द्वारा आत्मज्ञान प्राप्त करने के विषय पर प्रकाश डाला गया है। प्रत्येक भाग में ग्यारह सूत्र वाली तथा ग्यारह भागों में सम्पूर्ण यह पुस्तक स्त्री-पुरुष दोनों के लिए कल्याणकारी हो तथा जगत में सन्तुलन और शान्ति लाये।

This brings to an end the last Part of *The Kamasutra for Women* on sexuality and spirituality. May the eleven Parts of this book containing eleven sutras each help both women and men in bringing about harmony and peace in the cosmos.

Concluding Remarks

Draupadi is one of the principal female characters of the *Mahabharata*, the great epic from ancient India. Draupadi had five husbands; this happened, it is said, because in her previous life she had prayed to Lord Shiva for a husband who was the best archer and the bravest, most righteous, most cultured, and most beautiful of all men in the world. Lord Shiva, realizing that the limitations of human beings made Draupadi's wish impossible, blessed her with five separate husbands, each embodying one of the qualities requested. Despite her five exceptional men, Draupadi did not escape the pains and perils of life. The most righteous husband lost her while gambling in a game of chess, and the cousins of her husbands who had won her in this game subjected her to bitter humiliation. In the end, she lost all her five sons in the big war that erupted between the two clans.

As the story of Draupadi illustrates, real happiness does not lie in being matched with one or even several of the "best" men in the world. Happiness lies within and is attained only with inner peace and harmony. Peace comes with satisfaction; desire for more and more invariably leads to frustration, grief, and disharmony. A desire to stay in a given moment of time or to have things as they "used to be" leads to unhappiness. To dwell on an unpleasant experience makes it impossible to appreciate the pleasant aspects of life.

As for sexuality and companionship with men, women must proceed with an open and liberal mind. While common values and compatibility are essential for a long-term sexual relationship, it is not necessary to seek or desire sexual sharing with all the men one admires or enjoys being with. I say this not from any social or moral point of view but with the idea of one's personal satisfaction and happiness. A woman's ability to develop relationships with men at various levels can help her to lead a wholesome life. The same applies to men regarding relationships with women. Do not make yourself vulnerable and make sexuality your weakness; rather, share it with a conscious and aware mind and with a sense of responsibility for the other.

We must have faith in basic human goodness and not linger on past experiences. A bad father or a negative experience with a lover need not shake your faith in the rest of the men in the world. "All" men do not behave the same. Learn to observe others in a neutral manner. Our past experiences should enrich, not impoverish, us. If your "bad" experiences seem to repeat themselves, then perhaps it is time to examine what you may be contributing to the negative outcome.

Nobody in this world is indispensable, and life will go on even when we are no longer here. Some people dwell on the thought of what they cannot get, such as their dream man or woman. They attribute so much more to this person than he or she actually is that they linger their entire lives within these thoughts and imaginings. Such people are unable to enjoy the given moment. Remember that living on what was or was not, what would be or would have been, is the most detrimental thing you can do to yourself.

My purpose in discussing all these points is to develop a larger consciousness for all aspects of sexuality. However, there are many social dimensions of these problems that cannot be treated here in detail. In countries where women cannot open a bank account or get a room in a hotel or drive a vehicle, this book may seem like a fairytale. Women in these situations must use their strength to organize and raise their joint voice against such restrictions. I feel that even in such extreme situations, aggressive and reactionary methods do not bring fruitful results for women, men, or society as a whole. It is no doubt true that all men will not cooperate in creating a new social order, but neither will all women. Radical changes are always brought about by a handful of people. Besides, it is a ridiculous idea to think that women are exploited only by men. Whether it is at a sexual or a social level, the exploitation of women by women has proven to be no less.[1]

It may seem to the reader from my comments in Sutra 8 of Part II that I am against the institution of marriage. Rather, I believe that any institution or organization or value system which does not evolve with the changing times degenerates. We do not need to abandon the system of marriage, but we need to change the rigidity of the norms attached to it and make them more contemporary.

In Part II, I put forward a theory of the male–female ratio which is based upon the three fundamental qualities of the Cosmic Substance. This theory helps us see men and women in their primordial nature, free from the norms or values attached to them by different societies of the world. The theory of the three qualities of the Cosmic Substance has meaning only in a universal context, and though it stems from an Indian cultural tradition, it transcends the limits of that tradition. I feel this theory of a male–female nature in an ever-changing interdependent, interrelated cosmos allows for large variability within the two sexes and does not compartmentalize them. Such compartmentalization, imposed by social and religious systems, has had a very damaging effect throughout human history. When half the persons in a given society are subjected to injustice, the imbalance leads to the unhappiness of all. Think of all those countries where women are not even allowed to get out of their houses on their own and have to cover themselves from head to foot.

It is basic human nature to protect ourselves against injustice and an inner human need to maintain a minimum of freedom. Those who are subjected to injustice must fight against it by direct, indirect, or subtle means, depending upon the circumstances. When the extent of their fight is limited by their lack of freedom, women adopt dubious methods. They develop vindictive behavior and take their revenge on their children or other women. In many women subjected to injustice, negative traits such as stubbornness, jealousy, anger, fraudulence, and malice become prevalent—and it is the observation of this dimension of women which led some ancient writers to describe these characteristics as basic traits of women.

Some may question why it is so essential to have a smooth flow of sexual energy and what importance it has beyond pure physical pleasure. My own belief is that when sexual energy is hindered or suppressed, it often blocks other energy channels and may cause illness of one sort or another. (Some holistic physicians think that the increasing rate of breast and uterine cancer in women is due to a blockage of sexual expression.) My writing about methods of rejuvenation after delivery or ways of curing lack of sexual secretions or various yogic practices to enhance sexual expression are not meant as mere prescriptions for finding the "joy of sex."

The body is the field of all worldly activities. Whether these are material or spiritual gains, the body is the medium for all. Sexuality, one of the major activities of our bodies, serves not only procreation but sharing and communication between the two diverse forces of the universe. It seems that, by and large, the human race has been greatly mystified by sexuality. Many religions and cultures deny it as an important aspect of life. Yet its suppression always leads to crimes, perversions, mental disorders, and many other ailments. Reacting to this denial with flagrant sexual acting out then converts this holy natural phenomenon into vulgarity and obscenity. Through it all, women and children suffer most.

The hope for and solution to this multifarious problem lies in taking a cosmic view of sexuality, as free as possible from the culturally imposed norms and values. I believe that the fundamental principles are beyond space and time, that the appropriate expression of sexual energy can lead to a spiritual experience, and that we human beings should not leave this immense source of energy un-tapped within us. Sexual energy should never be suppressed. As a great sage of our times, the Dalai Lama, says:

> *I am sometimes asked whether this vow of celibacy is really desirable and indeed whether it is really possible. Suffice to say that its practice is not simply a matter of suppressing sexual desires. On the contrary, it is necessary fully to accept the existence of these desires and to transcend them by the power of reasoning. When successful, the results on the mind can be very beneficial. . . . The gratification of sexual desire can only ever give temporary satisfaction.*[2]

OM SHANTI

U.S. Sources for Ayurvedic and Homeopathic Ingredients

Sources for Herbs

The following list was compiled by the publisher for the reader's information and does not indicate a recommendation for the products of any particular source over another.

Kalustyan's
123 Lexington Avenue
New York, NY 10016
Tel: (212) 685-3451
Fax: (212) 683-8458

Spices, nuts, dried fruits, grains, beans, Eastern specialties

Retail and mail-order shop. Located in one of Manhattan's "little India" neighborhoods, around Lexington Avenue in the upper 20s.

Bazaar of India Imports, Inc.
1810 University Avenue
Berkeley, CA 94703-1516
Tel: (800) 261-SOMA [261-7662]
Fax: (510) 548-1115

Ayurvedic herbs, teas, books, essential oils, and other products

Mail-order shop.

Jean's Greens
RR 1 Box 55J, Hale Road
Rensselaerville, New York 12147
Tel. & Fax: (518) 239-TEAS [239-8327]

Herbs, teas, spices, essential oils, base oils, herbal products for face and body (Western herbs emphasized)

Mail-order shop.

> Osaanwin Herb Apothecary
> 112 Main Street, PO Box 964
> Montpelier, VT 05601
> Tel.: (802) 223-0888

Extensive herb selection, including Ayurvedic and culinary spices

Mail-order and retail shop.

Homeopathic Suppliers

> Arrowroot Standard Direct
> 83 East Lancaster Ave.
> Paoli, PA 19301
> Tel.: (800) 234-8879

Also carries Ayurvedic herbs

Mail-order and retail shop.

> Standard Homeopathic Company
> PO Box 61607
> Los Angeles, CA 90061
> Tel.: (800) 624-9659

Mail-order shop.

> Washington Homeopathic Pharmacy
> 4914 Del Ray Ave.
> Bethesda, MD 20814
> Tel.: (800) 336-1695

Mail-order shop.

> Boiron-Borneman
> Box 54
> Norwood, PA 19074
> Tel.: (800) BLU-TUBE [258-8823]

Notes

Preface

1. For details of these concepts, refer to my book *Yoga Sutra of Patanjali: A Scientific Exposition* (New Delhi: Clarion Books, 1996).

2. A. L. Basham, *The Wonder That Was India* (London: Fontana Books, 1971), p. 172.

3. *Atharva Veda*, IX (2), 19, 21.

4. Vinod Verma, *Yoga Sutra of Patanjali*.

Part I • Self-Awareness

1. For more details on this theme, see Carolyn Merchant, *Death of Nature* (New York: Harper & Row, 1980).

2. *Charaka Samhita*, "Sutrasthana," XI, 3–6.

Part II • Harmony in Male and Female Principles

1. The reader should try to understand the concept of equilibrium of the three qualities by understanding their different levels. For example, the stillness achieved through meditation is also opposite to movement, but it is not tamas, as this experience is at another level than the stillness which results from sleep. The experience of sleep is at the bodily level, and the activity of the mind continues during this time, whereas stillness achieved by meditation is the state when the activities of the mind come to a stop. This latter happens at an entirely different level which is beyond the bodily experience and is spiritual.

2. The word *meditation*, or *samadhi*, has a very specific sense in the present context. It is the last of the three stages of the mind after attain-

ing a thought-free state. For more details on this subject, see *Yoga Sutra of Patanjali* (Preface, note 1).

Part III • Menstruation and Sexuality

1. These tables and figures are from my books on Ayurveda (see *n2* and *Ayurveda for Life: Nutrition, Sexual Energy and Healing* [York Beach, Me.: Samuel Weiser, 1997]).

2. For more information on Ayurveda, see my book *Ayurveda: A Way of Life* (York Beach, Me.: Samuel Weiser, 1995).

3. Cress seeds contain some derivatives of estrogens, which are present in the volatile oils of the seeds. Therefore, for medicinal purposes, the seeds should not be more than a year old.

Part IV • Pregnancy, Childbirth, and Sexuality

1. For more details, refer to my book *Ayurveda: A Way of Life* (York Beach, Me.: Samuel Weiser, 1995).
2. *Charaka Samhita,* "*Shariarasthanam,*" III, 9.
3. For more details, refer to *Ayurveda for Life: Nutrition, Sexual Energy and Healing* (York Beach, Me.: Samuel Weiser, 1997).
4. *Charaka Samhita,* "*Shariarasthanam,*" IV, 9.

Part V • The Three Dimensions of a Woman

1. For a detailed discussion of this theme, see F. Capra, *The Turning Point*, New York: Bantam, 1984.
2. This figure is based on that in my book *Ayurveda for Work Efficiency* (in press).

Part VI • Physical Power and Sexuality

1. For more details, refer to my *Ayurveda: A Way of Life* (York Beach, Me.: Samuel Weiser, 1995), 128–129.
2. *Rig Veda,* I (3), 25–27.
3. *Yoga for Integral Health* contains a nine-week course for making the body gradually flexible and supple. Refer to this book also for the eightfold yogic practices.
4. *Yoga for Integral Health* also contains a valuable initiation into pranayama.

Part VIII • Atmosphere, Rituals, and Sexuality

1. In *Manusmriti*, a treatise on social code and conduct written by Manu a little before the Christian era, a contrary idea to this sutra has been expressed: "A woman does not examine a man's appearance, nor does she see other circumstances; whether ugly or beautiful, considering it is a man, she has carnal pleasure with him" (IX, 14).

   Manu adds that it is a natural phenomenon in women to desire coitus as soon as they see a man. Women have restless minds, they lack stability in love; therefore, the men should guard them to protect them. Beds, comfortable seats, jewelry, sexual desire, anger, fraudulence, malice, and bad behavior have been made for women by the Creator (IX, 17). The author also believes that a woman acquires the good or bad personality of the man she is married to and becomes just like him, as the river loses its identity after it merges into the sea (IX, 23).

   However, the author of the *Manusmriti* contradicts himself when he states that women bring fortune to men, they are worth worshipping because they give birth to offspring, they are the light of the household, and so on (IX, 26).

   All this shows that Manu had no clear views on the subject, and perhaps his writings depict his personal ambivalence and conflict.

2. *Kamasutra of Vatsyayana*, III, 2.

3. A. Mookerji and M. Khanna, *The Tantric Way* (Boston: New York Graphic Society, 1977); Agehananda Bharati, *The Tantric Tradition* (London: Rider, 1965).

4. There are many methods to achieve singlepointedness of the mind. Different schools follow different methods. There are gurus and guides who initiate people on this path. Religions of the world teach this one way or the other. The practice of breathing allied to concentration is fundamental to many martial arts of the world. I have tried to explain everything in a simple manner and have made an effort to develop easy methods so that you are able to learn on your own. You may have a guru or guide, but ultimately it is your own efforts which lead you to achieve stillness of mind and singlepointedness (generally called meditation). Gurus can only show the way, but the achievement of the aim lies in strong determination and persistence of the adept. That is why it is repeatedly said that your practice may be only for six minutes a day, but you must exercise very day.

Part IX • Rhythm and Variety in Sexuality

1. For the Salutation to the Sun exercises, see my *Ayurveda: A Way of Life* (York Beach, Me.: Samuel Weiser, 1995).

Part X • Rejuvenation and Aphrodisiacs

1. *Rig Veda*, X, 129.4
2. Alain Daniélou, *The Gods of India—Hindu Polytheism* (New York: Inner Tradition International, 1985), p. 16.

   Note: The reader should understand that *linga* (phallus), the symbol of Shiva and of the male principle, is always shown in *yoni* (the female sex organ), the symbol of the female principle (see Part VIII, Fig. 29). Together, they show the unification and oneness of the two principles, which is the cause of the phenomenal world.
3. *Yogatattva Upanishad*, I, 31.
4. For more details of the inner cleansing methods, see my *Ayurveda: A Way of Life* (York Beach, Me.: Samuel Weiser, 1995) pp. 91–103.
5. For more details on the subject see original Ayurvedic texts such as *Charaka Samhita, Sushurata Samhita, Sarangadhara Samhita*, etc.
6. *Charaka Samhita, Chikitsasthanam*, II (1), 50–51.

Concluding Remarks

1. Although many professionial women grumble that they cannot progress because of male domination, a large number of women have told me that they have had their worst experiences with other women. I feel that often those who blame men do not truly excel in their professions, and by blaming the other sex, they save themselvs from facing the real situation. Whether we are men or women, we must struggle hard in this competitive world.

   Woman's exploitation of woman is an age-old practice seen in prostitution run by women, in the abuse of mothers-in-law in many parts of the world, in many women's obsessive desire to have male children, and so on. Even in the Western world, highly educated parents often do not encourage their daughters to attend professional schools, although they insist it is necessary for their sons to do so. The daughters of doctors or executives often end up as technicians or secretaries.
2. *Freedom in Exile: The Autobiography of the Dalai Lama* (New York: HarperCollins, 1991), p. 225.